How Stress Works

How Stress Works

Understanding the New Science of
Stress Hormones

DR RICHARD MACKENZIE AND PETER WALKER

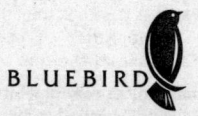

BLUEBIRD

First published 2025
This edition published 2026 by Bluebird
an imprint of Pan Macmillan
The Smithson, 6 Briset Street, London EC1M 5NR
EU representative: Macmillan Publishers Ireland Ltd, 1st Floor,
The Liffey Trust Centre, 117–126 Sheriff Street Upper,
Dublin 1 D01 YC43
Associated companies throughout the world

ISBN 978-1-0350-4904-2

Copyright © Richard Mackenzie and Peter Walker 2025

This book aims to provide helpful general information on the subjects that it addresses. It is not in any way a substitute for the advice of the reader's own doctor(s) or other medical professionals based on the reader's own individual conditions, symptoms or concerns. If the reader needs personal medical, health, dietary, exercise or other assistance or advice, the reader should consult a competent doctor and/or other qualified health care professionals. The reader is advised not to undertake, cease or modify any treatments, diets or health procedures without consulting a professional. The publisher and authors specifically disclaim responsibility for any liability that may result from the use of information contained in this book.

The rights of Richard Mackenzie and Peter Walker to be identified as the authors of this work have been asserted by them in accordance with the Copyright, Designs and Patents Act 1988.

All rights reserved. No part of this publication may be reproduced, stored in a retrieval system, or transmitted, in any form, or by any means (including, without limitation, electronic, mechanical, photocopying, recording or otherwise) without the prior written permission of the publisher.

Pan Macmillan does not have any control over, or any responsibility for, any author or third-party websites (including, without limitation, URLs, emails and QR codes) referred to in or on this book.

1 3 5 7 9 8 6 4 2

A CIP catalogue record for this book is available from the British Library.

Typeset by Six Red Marbles UK, Thetford, Norfolk

Printed and bound in the UK using 100% Renewable Electricity by CPI Group (UK) Ltd

This book is sold subject to the condition that it shall not, by way of trade or otherwise, be lent, hired out, or otherwise circulated without the publisher's prior consent in any form of binding or cover other than that in which it is published and without a similar condition including this condition being imposed on the subsequent purchaser. The publisher does not authorize the use or reproduction of any part of this book in any manner for the purpose of training artificial intelligence technologies or systems. The publisher expressly reserves this book from the Text and Data Mining exception in accordance with Article 4(3) of the European Union Digital Single Market Directive 2019/790.

Visit **www.panmacmillan.com/bluebird** to read more
about all our books and to buy them.

Contents

CHAPTER 1 A NEW UNDERSTANDING OF STRESS — 1

CHAPTER 2 A SHORT HISTORY OF STRESS — 15

CHAPTER 3 THE HORMONES THAT SHAPE YOUR LIFE — 32

CHAPTER 4 THE NEED FOR HOMEOSTASIS — 51

CHAPTER 5 STRESS, STATUS AND WORK — 71

CHAPTER 6 CARBOHYDRATES, APPETITES AND STIGMA: Stress and Weight — 94

CHAPTER 7 THE TIDAL WAVE OF ILLNESS: Stress and Diabetes — 116

CHAPTER 8 THE DELICATE BALANCE: How Stress Can Affect Fertility — 138

CHAPTER 9 LOVE, TOUCH AND INHERITANCE: Early Years and Stress — 153

CHAPTER 10 ROUTES OUT OF STRESS — 176

Epilogue: A Light in the Mist — 201
Acknowledgements — 207
Notes — 209
About the Authors — 225

CHAPTER 1

A New Understanding of Stress

We are now approaching a century since the word 'stress' acquired its current usage, having been used originally only in physics and engineering to describe the way force is exerted on physical objects. It's also more than forty years since 'stressed out' entered the lexicon. These days, it's fair to say, everyone knows what it means. Or do they? It is a word we're all familiar with and yet the closer you look, the more slippery it can sometimes feel.

If someone came up and asked, 'Are you stressed?', for many people the short answer would be a simple 'Yes' – if perhaps not at that exact moment, then in a broader sense, most definitely. This, at least, is what the studies and surveys show us. Three quarters of British adults say that at least once over the last year they have been sufficiently stressed that they felt overwhelmed or unable to cope.[1] But others might reply: it depends what you mean. Stress is many things. Most of all, it is elastic, elusive, a term with a firm basis in academic research that can nonetheless only be measured subjectively. Despite stress having a long and ever-evolving history, one constant is that it has always been arguably as much a cultural phenomenon as a scientific one.

Over the decades, many hundreds of books have been written about stress and how to cope with it. Some have sold extraordinarily well and become highly influential. Yet it's fair to say that things don't seem to be getting much better. An estimated 2.8 million Britons cannot work due to long-term sickness, with over half of this total estimated to be due to stress and related conditions like anxiety and depression.[2] Two of the other main reasons why people say they are unable to hold down jobs, type 2 diabetes and chronic pain, are increasing at pandemic-like speed and, crucially, are linked at least in part to stress.

Nowadays, we fret about the stresses of screen-based home employment, or jobs taken by artificial intelligence. A hundred and fifty years ago, anguished Victorian writers feared that the human mind was not equipped to deal with advances like 70mph travel on steam trains, or instant long-distance communication via the telegraph.

Why another book? While stress can't be 'solved', we are approaching a thrilling new era of understanding stress as a phenomenon, both medically and in broader terms, and therefore discovering ways it can be mitigated. Researchers are increasingly able to explain stress as a biological-societal construct. What happens in our body does not exist in isolation; it is almost always moulded, often very significantly, by the external circumstances we face, many of which are entirely beyond our control.

This book will not present stress as something to be vanquished through a list of individual action points, ones which invariably end up proving so impractical they leave the reader feeling guilty and, yes, more stressed. Stress is part of our lives. It is something that cannot be measured by a test, or plotted as a series of numbers on a graph. It is real but also entirely personal. There are no one-size-fits-all answers.

This is not a self-help book, although we hope it is a book which could help many people. The better we understand how and why stress occurs, and how it impacts our physical and mental well-being, the more we can do about it. This is a much bigger picture than you might think.

What *is* Stress?

Near the end of his academic career, the bulk of it devoted to studying stress, the American psychologist Seymour Levine said he had not only lost count of the number of conferences regarding stress he had attended, but also the number of times a participant at one of those conferences argued that 'stress' in its current meaning should be dropped in favour of something more precise.

In popular use, and sometimes even in academia, stress is a word that can simultaneously mean the input – the stimuli that create stress, whether external or internal – as well as the body's reaction to these things, both immediately and over the medium or long term.

Hans Selye, the researcher who popularized the definition of stress in its modern usage, also coined the term 'stressor', something which creates stress, to distinguish it from the reaction. Useful though this is in some ways, it still leaves you with a definition for stressor as nothing more than 'something that causes stress'. It can all feel a bit circular.

Some experts have tried to define stressors as stimuli which disturb, or potentially disturb, what is known as homeostasis, a healthy body's self-balancing system for complex internal systems like blood sugars. This is, however, both a bit technical and also slightly undermined by the fact that definitions differ as to what actually constitutes homeostasis.

Perhaps the best compromise is a fairly generalized definition, like this one taken from a weighty academic book about stress, which defines it as 'a real or interpreted threat to the physiological or psychological integrity of an individual that results in physiological and/or behavioural responses',[3] with the optional add-on that this biological response elevates the person's levels of stress-connected hormones.

> That will do us for now. When this book refers to 'stress', that is broadly what we mean. But do remember, the fact it is such a flexible concept means that if you feel something in your life is a stress, no one can tell you it isn't. To your body this is an entirely personal matter, and rightly so.

Hormones: the chemical messengers

The science of hormones, officially known as endocrinology, is still fairly new. The very word 'hormone' was only created in 1905, borrowed from *ormao*, a classical Greek verb meaning to arouse or excite. It was in 1936 that Hans Selye, the hugely industrious Hungarian-Canadian researcher who introduced us to 'stress' in its modern parlance, developed and popularized the idea that the condition and its physical ill effects are hormonal in nature.[4]

Hormones are, at their simplest, internally secreted chemical messengers which carry biological signals through the bloodstream to the particular organs they target. At the time Selye made his breakthrough, just a handful had been properly identified. Scientists have subsequently isolated more than fifty, many released from eight glands scattered across the body from the head to the groin and influencing everything from mood, sleep and our immune system, to sexual desire, puberty and growth. When it comes to stress, the key players are catecholamines, the collective term for the likes of adrenaline and noradrenaline, which kick-start our heart-pumping, prehistoric 'fight or flight' response, and then cortisol, which brings another, longer-lasting surge of energy from stored bodily sugars, and about which we will hear a lot more in this book.

While there are evolutionary benefits to this hormonal alarm system – it exists in all mammals, not to mention in birds, fish, amphibians and reptiles – the problem for contemporary humans is that our lives have changed beyond recognition while our hormonal response has not. The crucial difference is that modern stress is generally not a one-off, but a long-running sequence of events.

We still occasionally face the sort of stressful situation that would have been familiar to an early human, even if this might now mean immediate and existential peril from a speeding car rather than, say, a snarling wolf. But in modern life, such genuinely life-or-death situations are rare. These days, when we experience a sudden rush of stress-released hormones, it is almost always a response to a threat which, to our wolf-confronting ancestor, might seem minimal. It could be a worrying large electricity bill, a difficult meeting at work, perhaps anxieties that a parent is becoming frail, or a child is unhappy.

There is a crucial point to note here. While none of those stresses is going to kill you, that does not mean they are not real. The resulting influx of hormones is the same, as is their effect on your body. And this impact can be significant. Stress can hugely deplete your mental and physical resources. This is all the more so given modern stress is so often a cascade of occurrences, some of which might, on their own, feel minor. Stress presents most intensely as an accumulative condition, one that builds up, often only half noticed until the tipping point is reached. It is the repetition that is key, both from the perspective of its sheer inexorableness, and also because of the way the endlessly-repeated surge of hormones can take a toll on the body.

Much of this long-term bodily impact is related to insulin, the hormone central to processing blood sugars, which works less efficiently in a stressed body. Regular, inescapable stress is very often a path towards something known as insulin resistance, where your body starts to respond less well to insulin, meaning it becomes less effective at removing sugars from your bloodstream, a crucial part of your body's self-sustaining balance. Insulin resistance is itself often the precursor to type 2 diabetes, the lifestyle-related variant of the chronic condition in which the body is unable to properly process such sugars. Type 2 diabetes is now so common it is arguably the biggest single contributor to long-term sickness in modern life, as we shall see in detail in Chapter 7.

Luckily, this is not just a story of gloom. New techniques and innovative research are allowing scientists to track the path towards insulin resistance at a cellular level, and perhaps one day to understand how it might be stopped, or delayed. Even now, there are new insights about the way hormones interact with our body which allow people to mitigate the physical repercussions of stress, some which are far from obvious. One example, as we shall see in Chapter 6, new research suggests that large amounts of high-intensity exercise can actually elevate levels of stress hormones, making it harder for some people to lose weight. Stress might be ubiquitous, but it is not always straightforward.

All that said, even a complete understanding of the interactions of every single hormone would not make sense without the context of outside factors, ones which prompt our bodies to secrete hormones in greater or lesser amounts and with greater or lesser regularity. We do not exist in a laboratory. The real world makes daily and unpredictable demands on our endocrine systems, and no one reacts in precisely the same way.

Stress is personal

Michael Marmot is one of the world's most respected authorities on health-based inequalities. Earlier in his career, spanning more than half a century, he helped make a key breakthrough about the societal context of stress, discovering that its most serious physical manifestations are not largely a problem for the managerial class, as then popularly believed, but tend to be worse the lower down you are on the social scale.

Marmot can recall the moment he first truly understood the inseparable link between the lives people lead and the mental and physical health they have to deal with. As a medical student shadowing a psychiatrist in Sydney, he saw a female outpatient who felt lethargic and could not sleep. Asked for more details, the woman explained that her husband was abusive, her son was in prison and her teenage daughter was pregnant.

The psychiatrist's response, Marmot recounts, was to suggest she switch from one type of prescription tranquillizer to another. The idea that a change in medication might solve her very obviously life-based problems was, Marmot recalls with pointed understatement, 'not compelling.'[5]

Stress is still viewed as a largely medicalized affair, or else a type of individual struggle, in both cases separate from the actual lives people lead. If there is one single message to take away from this book it is the fact that stress is not someone's 'fault', or responsibility, a thing to feel guilty about. To begin with, stress can sometimes be of use. As well as the miraculously head-clearing and muscle-enabling properties of a rush of adrenaline as that hypothetical car (or wolf) heads towards you, the same hormonal response can sometimes be necessary in less dramatic circumstances. Some studies have shown stress can even improve memory function in some instances, a boon for the pressured student.

Once again we return to the vital difference between a one-off or short-term stressor, and stress as a chronic condition. This is where Marmot's long-ago patient comes in. She exemplified the way that stress, and the hormonal build-up which comes with it, is almost always imposed by external factors which are themselves almost always beyond our control, and in many cases due to societal structures such as poverty and inequality. Reams of studies have demonstrated that you are statistically more likely to experience stress if you are poor, or if you are a woman, or from a minority ethnic background, or are disabled. Too many guides to stress neglect this fundamental and inescapable framing.

Such personal circumstances, including our childhoods, greatly shape our response to the stress we experience, which in turn affects our health. When it comes to the chance of developing stress-connected ailments like type 2 diabetes, other factors are also important, notably diet and activity levels. But even here, context is vital. Study after study has shown that if you expose people artificially to stress and then present them with a menu of food choices, they invariably gravitate towards less healthy and more caloric options than do those in a control group not put through the same stressful experience. Similarly, reams of parallel academic papers have demonstrated that when people are stressed they tend to live more sedentary lives. Everything is connected.

The cumulative effects of all this on public health can be startling. Researchers have calculated that if you take the Jubilee underground line eastwards in London, average male life expectancy drops by about one year per stop between Westminster and Canning Town, as incomes in the surrounding areas decline and inequalities increase.[6] In the UK's wealthiest areas, people can expect nearly twenty more years of healthy life than in the most deprived.[7]

Such disparities are both a product of existing stress and the creator of more of it. Stress, particularly financial stress, tends to be self-perpetuating. One fascinating US study stopped people in a shopping mall and asked them to consider one of two entirely hypothetical financial situations, involving a car repair costing either $150 or $1,500. These 'easy' and 'hard' financial scenarios were allocated randomly to the participants, who after thinking about the car repair were then given a cognitive task to complete. Finally, they were questioned about their family income. The results showed that after musing over the cheaper car-repair option, the poorer and richer participants performed similarly in the cognitive test. But when the $1,500 repair was on people's minds, poorer participants fared notably worse. Even thinking about a bill, not one they had to pay, clouded their thinking.[8]

Other experiments have delved into why people on lower incomes tend to, on average, deal less well with things like completing a course of medication, or cooking healthy food. The conclusion is that stress from unpaid bills and suchlike can create a type of tunnel vision, sometimes known as a 'scarcity mindset', which makes it much harder to focus on other, less immediate tasks. Studies have quantified these effects variously as being about the same as losing an entire night of sleep, being a chronic alcoholic rather than a non-drinker, or suddenly shedding close to fifteen IQ points.[9] This is not a minor impact.

The second link between stress and circumstance is perhaps even more vital: not everyone deals with stress the same way. People can experience near-identical challenges and find that they produce very different levels of cortisol, and that their bodies are affected by the cortisol to very different degrees. As we shall see in Chapter 9, much of this comes down to the early stages of life and in particular its very start, even before birth. Numerous studies have shown that a mother's exposure to consistently high cortisol during pregnancy tends to make their child less able to deal with the physiological manifestations of stress when they are an adult.

One fascinating project showed that when a group of young university students were asked to look at pictures of faces with angry expressions, those whose parents came from a lower social standing showed a bigger reaction in their amygdala, the mysterious and tiny part of the brain that processes emotions and in turn tells other parts of the brain when we are under threat.[10] This sort of 'neural embedding', as researchers term it, is largely unconscious and therefore very difficult to even know about, let alone escape.

Fight, flight and cortisol

These seemingly inescapable differences in how we cope with stress come back to the ancient fight-or-flight response, and a particular element of it, something called the hypothalamic-pituitary-adrenal axis, or the HPA axis for short, named after the section of the brain and the two sets of glands which are involved. Such technical terms can feel daunting, but the process is in fact quite straightforward. And it is, in many ways, the very centre of this book's story.

When our hypothetical cave-dweller, or their contemporary loft-apartment-living equivalent, faces sudden danger, the stress response is so rapid that before the conscious brain has even processed that a threat exists, the first wave of emergency hormones, adrenaline and noradrenaline, are already pumping around the body. These increase the pulse rate and raise the blood pressure, making them alert and primed to react. It is an all-body operation, including the notably prehistoric phenomenon of piloerection, the term for hairs standing on end, a throwback to our more hairy past when doing so would both help to trap heat and make us look bigger to an aggressor. Goose pimples are simply the hair-free element of this process.

Now the red-alert response has done its thing, the HPA axis begins a second wave of hormonal response, flooding the body with cortisol. In evolutionary terms, cortisol's role is similarly hugely useful, prompting a more sustained surge of energy from stored glucose. If adrenaline was there to shock our ancestor into shouting at the wolf so it backed off, the cortisol-released glucose would assist with a sprint away from danger. What should then happen is that another element of our involuntary nervous system, known as the parasympathetic nervous system, dials down this hormonal response. But in too many people, this hormonal brake doesn't fully engage, and the cortisol keeps on flowing.

Cortisol is, in absolute terms, a mere drop in our systems, with the average person producing slightly under 10 milligrams per day, perhaps slightly over a tenth of a million of their body mass. But in terms of our health, even our life destiny, it punches very much above its weight. Cortisol is central to many of our bodily rhythms. And when it gets knocked out of alignment, so do they.

While adrenaline is usually only released in response to urgent stress, cortisol has a role beyond its emergency function. In smaller quantities it emerges in waves over the course of the day, acting almost like a hormonal alarm clock. For a healthy person, natural cortisol levels rise gradually during the night to a morning peak, typically between about 6 a.m. and 8 a.m., to help get us out of bed, and then decline into the afternoon and evening.

This is a pattern that can be easily disturbed. A visceral fight-or-flight situation can see the amount of cortisol in your body multiply by ten times or even more. But even everyday worries and concerns, especially if repeated, can trigger a cortisol response, making the body believe it needs a mass of blood sugar when it does not. This reaction becomes cumulative and eventually chronic, meaning people are walking around with cortisol levels that are permanently higher than they should be. This brings a mass of health risks, many connected to the way cortisol impedes the work of insulin, including the potential to develop diabetes, weight gain, higher blood pressure, heart disease and other ailments, not to mention a greater likelihood of depression, anxiety and poor sleep.

The good news is that our understanding of all this is moving at pace, helped in part by new methods to monitor hormones. Where once cortisol could only be measured using laborious blood samples, this can now be done from saliva, with self-administered swabs helping researchers understand why it ebbs and flows over a day. Other methods are emerging which could, in effect, bring real-time cortisol monitoring. One option is for wearable patches that measure it via sweat. A still more science-fiction-style proposal is a Korean project to develop what would in effect be a wireless-transmitting contact lens, which would monitor cortisol concentrations in tears and report back.[11]

Your authors

It might now be time for a bit of context. This is a co-authored book, so who are we, and why should you trust us to guide you through this new world of stress? The first point to note is that this is a joint production. Throughout almost all the book, both of us authors are speaking, as it were. Where there are occasional digressions into individual ideas or narratives, we make it plain who is doing it.

Richard is a university academic specializing in insulin resistance and how stress affects the body. He also leads on such disorders at a Harley Street clinic, seeing people at the front line of how all this interacts. Peter is a journalist and writer, officially covering politics, who has written two other books with a health focus. He has a particular interest in health inequalities and the way these are affected by society and by political decisions. As you will hopefully see, this dual focus helps to place stress in a wider context, offering opportunities to both understand it as a phenomenon and potentially cope with its impact.

It is Richard's clinical work which is relevant here. Now that we have explained the science behind how increased cortisol can affect the body, it's time to show a real-life example. And it is real life: every one of the case studies in this book is based on an actual person. However, details have been altered or otherwise anonymized. If you think you actually know any of the people described, you are mistaken.

Ruth's story

This brings us to Ruth, who is an exemplar of how the stress response can be provoked into running unchecked, and what happens when it does. Now forty-six, Ruth grew up amid a certain amount of emotional chaos, a good part of it triggered after her father died suddenly when she was three and her younger sister was one. Her mother raised the girls but struggled with alcohol and her emotions. The trio were close, if combustible. As an adult, Ruth has faced periods of depression and anxiety. Both of these can be experienced by people who are not stressed, but they very often come together – studies have shown that around half of people newly diagnosed with depression have elevated cortisol levels. She has a responsible job as an administration manager for a law firm, but finds the pace difficult and worries that she takes more time off sick than her colleagues.

All this has exerted an understandable mental toll. In everyday life, Ruth seems confident and competent. But she would often spend her evening worrying about a work meeting the next day, or her sister's turbulent life. There was also a physical impact. Since she had been a teenager, Ruth had been above what is seen as a healthy weight. In her late thirties she was diagnosed with type 2 diabetes, as well as a form of intermittent inflammatory joint pain which makes physical activity harder. Ruth was in a long-term relationship for over a decade, but she and her partner were unable to conceive.

She came to Richard's clinic to have her blood glucose and insulin sensitivity tested, but also to learn about her cortisol levels. She had been reading about chronic stress and its impacts, and guessed this could be a factor in her various ailments. And this seemed to be the case. Cortisol tests are usually taken in the morning, when the flow is near its peak, and at 8 a.m. Ruth's reading was above the normal range. Her blood pressure was also higher than ideal, which she had not previously realized.

This was, it seemed, a textbook case of several decades of life history pointing in one direction. But, over time, some things changed. Ruth started psychotherapy, seeking to better understand elements of her story, notably her childhood and its impact on her. She read more about stress and how cortisol reactivity can be set from infancy. And she came to a decision: while rewriting the past to undo this was not possible, she could try to tackle its effects.

She agreed with her boss to start working four days a week, trying to use the extra time to connect more with her family and friends. Perhaps most crucially of all, she got a dog, and from living a largely sedentary life – she used to joke about driving the 400 metres to her local shop for milk – Ruth began walking longer and longer distances. As her fitness improved, she took up other exercise, including year-round outdoor swimming.

Ruth's cortisol is now lower, if still slightly above what would be considered ideal. She can find work stressful, but is more open with her boss and colleagues about this. Her weight has dropped slightly and her waist size is notably smaller, often a sign of improved health independently of the body mass index, or BMI. The biggest change has come in her blood glucose and insulin. With the extra physical activity, these are almost normal. Her type 2 diabetes is, in effect, in remission, to the delight of her family – and her doctor. Ruth's joints are still sometimes painful but notably less so. Her blood pressure is now well within healthy ranges.

This was not a miracle cure. If any book about stress does offer such a thing, you should probably put it straight back on the bookshop shelf. It must also be noted that Ruth's is a particular case and what worked for her will not necessarily do the same for others. Chronic stress is highly personal and very persistent. But it is also sufficiently broad and nuanced that it can be tackled on several fronts at once. For Ruth, this involved trying to understand why she is more susceptible than some other people and to feel less guilty about it, while simultaneously seeking to mitigate the ways her body expressed this in-built propensity.

Like Ruth, this book also has several intertwined hopes and aims. The first is to explain, authoritatively but engagingly, what stress is and how it has existed over time, as both a societal and medical concept. It will also explore the various ways it can affect your body and how this is very often shaped by lifetime experiences. Subsequent chapters deal with more specific related issues such as weight, diabetes and the potential impact on fertility, for both women and men. Finally, there are some ideas for ways people can try to understand the stress they face, feel and absorb, and to perhaps lessen some of these impacts.

To say it once again: this is not a self-help book. The world is already full of those. It is instead what you might call a guide, a route map to one of the most vexed, argued-over and ubiquitous phenomena of human life. And as with all stories, to understand where we are now, we first need a look to the past.

CHAPTER 2

A Short History of Stress

Stress has, very obviously, always existed. But as this chapter shows, the phenomenon in the way we broadly understand it today is surprisingly modern, in fact less than a century old. In this contemporary form, stress emerged more or less simultaneously from the research laboratory and within Western culture as a whole. This is not a history lesson for the sake of it – if you want to understand stress properly, you first have to know what it means.

The beginnings of this new era had a slightly low-key dawn: a university laboratory in Montreal in 1936, where Hans Selye, who we encountered briefly in Chapter 1, began injecting a series of unfortunate rats with toxic substances. Stress, and society as a whole, would never be quite the same again.

Selye was a vastly industrious Austrian–Hungarian doctor and research scientist who spent almost all his career in Canada, producing more than 1,700 academic articles and thirty-nine books. When it comes to stress, he is both a pivotal figure in its evolution and something of a contradiction. Selye's idea of 'general adaptation syndrome' more or less invented modern stress physiology, introducing the idea that a range of seemingly unconnected ailments are not just caused by long-term stress but, specifically, by the repeated and chronic triggering of the body's hormonal alarm system.

At the same time, Selye's laboratory work to support this was limited and, some critics argued, ultimately unconvincing. He spent the majority of his working life less as a discoverer of new concepts than a proselytizer of the one he had already devised, a tireless spokesman for his own era of stress. And despite his scientific impact, it is this latter role which is arguably more important.

As defined by Selye and his outriders, stress became a ubiquitous cultural phenomenon, beginning in North America before spreading globally. The idea that disseminated was heavily flavoured by individualism, a sense that this was a problem for people to cope with on their own, some faring better than others, rather than being a product of wider forces which might be challenged or changed. As such, it was heavily imbued with guilt for those who felt they had perhaps failed some sort of test.

Selye's was also an implicitly macho vision of chronic stress, helping to lay down the stereotype of a highly-paid, overworked male executive struggling with his stomach ulcers in a glass office, not an assembly-line worker toiling on the factory floor, let alone a woman trying to find the hours for childcare and domestic chores alongside a job.

This should not diminish the significance of Selye's breakthrough, or his extraordinary career. As a young researcher in the biochemistry department of Montreal's McGill University, Selye was tasked with trying to identify as-yet undiscovered female sex hormones by injecting rats with various extracts collected from cow ovaries, with the responses monitored before the rats were killed and dissected.

No matter what extract he used, Selye found the same physiological results: enlarged adrenal glands, damage to the lymphatic system – which plays a major role in the immune response – and peptic ulcers in the stomach and small intestine. Intrigued, he substituted the injections for deliberately stressful situations, for example placing the rats on the freezing-cold roof of the laboratory building in winter, or making them run for long periods on a treadmill. Once again, the physiological results were the same. This was starting to look like a pattern.

Selye was no ordinary academic. Born János Selye in Vienna, he spent his childhood in Komárom, a town which straddled the border of Hungary and what was then Czechoslovakia, before studying medicine and organic chemistry at Prague University. This upbringing at the confluence of so many cultures in the Austro-Hungarian empire meant that even as a young child Selye could speak four languages. After medical school he began a research career at Johns Hopkins University in the US before James Collip, the famed biochemist who was part of the Canadian team which isolated insulin in the early 1920s – one of the most significant medical discoveries of the century – sponsored Selye to come to McGill in 1932.

Pivotal to Selye's insight was his time as a medical student in Prague. In his best-selling book *The Stress of Life*, Selye recalled the moment in 1925 when he and his fellow trainee doctors had finished their theoretical learning and were shown a series of actual patients for the first time. 'What impressed me, the novice . . . was that so few signs and symptoms were actually characteristic of any one disease; most of the disturbances were apparently common to many, or perhaps even to all, diseases,' he wrote, saying this appeared to be a 'syndrome of just being sick'. When he explained this idea to the doctors, Selye recalled, he was laughed at.[1]

Selye's genius was to connect this slightly vague notion of a generalized ailment to the rats' uniform symptoms, whether from injections, cold, or being forced to run to exhaustion, and then to identify the crucial role of the body's hormonal response when exposed to destabilizing external factors, which he called stress. This modern usage of the word first got an airing in a 1935 paper by Selye about the rat experiments.[2] It was a year later that he tentatively explained his wider theory in a brief article – Selye counted it as '74 lines in a single column' – for the British journal *Nature*. This set out Selye's observation that the rats' biological response to what he termed 'nocuous agents', whether the injections or things like excessive cold or exercise, was always the same: an initial period of alarm, followed by what he named a 'resistance stage' and then, if the damaging external factor was maintained, by exhaustion and ultimately death.[3] He gave this process the slightly cryptic name of 'general adaptation syndrome'.

In his many dozens of subsequent papers and articles, this idea, which he sometimes called – a bit self-referentially – 'Selye's syndrome', was expanded into an all-encompassing mind-and-hormone concept of stress in which repeated or excessive triggering by external factors is linked to a series of diseases and ailments, not just the ulcers observed in rats, but also high blood pressure, asthma and some cancers. It was the repetition of stressors, the 'chronicity' in medical terms, that was key, plus the emphasis on the release of cortisol and other longer-acting hormones, not just the short blasts of adrenaline and noradrenaline in emergencies, as we saw in the opening chapter. This was, if scientifically imprecise at times, pretty much the same notion of chronic stress that we have today.

There are other fascinating details to Selye's early work. One is the theory for why the first set of rats, simply given injections rather than left on a frozen roof or placed on a treadmill, developed stereotypical stress symptoms. If Selye was a brilliant theoretical scientist, the story goes, he was notably less good at practical laboratory work. He was particularly inept at handling rats, meaning their ulcers were less a result of the hormonal extracts than the way he tended to squeeze them too tightly or drop them mid-jab, necessitating a frantic chase around the laboratory floor.

Another curiosity is his semantic gift to the world. However brilliant a polyglot, Selye was writing his articles in what was by then a fifth or sixth language, and when he chose 'stress' to explain his phenomenon he had no idea about its long-standing use in physics to denote forces acting on a physical material. In his first article for *Nature*, Selye also used 'alarm reaction', but worried that this too closely described just the first phase of his syndrome. One fellow academic who worked with Selye in later years heard him complain that 'had his knowledge of English been more precise, he would have gone down in history as the father of the "strain" concept.'[4]

In fairness to Selye, his definition was not too much of a linguistic leap. Taken from the Latin verb *stringere*, meaning to pull together tightly, when 'stress' first emerged in English around the fourteenth century it usually referred to a form of physical distress. This gradually evolved from denoting an external factor to an inner state, and even after its adoption in physics and engineering, by the nineteenth century a few writers used it to mean the medical consequences of prolonged physical hardship, not a huge distance from Selye's version. Either way, his definition stuck — and spread. In *The Stress of Life*, Selye describes giving a lecture in France and being unable to think of a useful French translation, so deciding to talk about *le stress*. As a noun it remains in French today, along with *der Stress* in German, *el estrés* in Spanish, *o estresse* in Portuguese, and so on.[5]

At the time of Selye's discovery in the 1930s, popular notions of stress, or whichever alternative term was used, were barely different from Victorian psychosomatic concepts like nerves, hysteria and the vapours. Exemplifying this nineteenth-century mode of thinking was George Miller Beard, a US doctor who specialized in problems of the nervous system, eventually coming up with a somewhat all-encompassing diagnosis he called neurasthenia.

Beard's idea, set out in his evocatively titled 1881 book *American Nervousness*, was that the human body has a finite amount of so-called nervous force, which, if used up, whether by worries or external factors, causes ailments including fatigue, high blood pressure and headaches.[6] Beard, who shared with Selye a keen ability to promote his own ideas, gave a dizzyingly long list of other possible symptoms of neurasthenia, including sore teeth, the tendency to avert one's eyes, or saying one word when you meant another. He also believed that the quantity of nervous force people began with was hereditary and that neurasthenia was primarily a problem for the well-off.

In a precursor to the cliché about stress being a result of the intolerable pace of modern life, Beard claimed that neurasthenia had never existed before his time and was also unknown in poorer countries. It was, he argued, caused by five contemporary and highly particular things: steam power; telegraph communications;

science; newspapers and magazines; and the 'mental activity of women'. Minor aggravating factors included dry air, civil and religious liberties, and 'the phenomenal beauty of the American girl of the highest type'.

Beard was viewed even by some contemporaries as a quack, and his theories were in some ways little more than a highbrow dressing-up of the sort of generalized worries about fatigue and anxiety used to advertise a multitude of 'nerve tonics' and proprietary tablets featuring ingredients ranging from iron to more alarming substances like strychnine or arsenic. Nonetheless, his era of stress and the new one introduced by Selye ran concurrently for a number of years. As late as the 1950s, newspapers ran advertisements for products like Phyllosan: 'To strengthen your Nerves and increase all your Physical and Vital forces'. The 1968 edition of the American Psychiatric Association's list of mental disorders still listed neurasthenia, albeit as just seventy-five words in a 136-page manual.[7] Things were, however, gradually starting to change. And as with many such social revolutions, war played its part.

The soldier's heart

War is a very obvious source of extreme stress, and even by the time Selye was devising his ideas it had already provided several insights, as well as an equal number of false starts. During the US Civil War, doctors identified something they called the 'soldier's heart', a propensity for troops to suffer palpitations and shortness of breath. In modern medicine these would be instantly recognized as likely symptoms of post-traumatic stress disorder; at the time it was blamed on physical overexertion, or the tightness of knapsack straps across men's chests.

Half a century later, when the phenomenon of shell shock was witnessed in the First World War, doctors initially assumed it was the result of brain injury from the blasts, even though many sufferers were physically unhurt. Others took a different view. William Rivers, the pioneering psychiatrist portrayed in Pat Barker's *Regeneration* trilogy of novels, treated shell-shocked officers, including the poet Siegfried Sassoon, with a talking-based regime influenced by Freud and psychoanalysis.

Selye was born in 1907 and thus had a ringside seat to the beginning of the century's chaos. He was eleven when the Austro-Hungarian empire, in which he lived with his Hungarian father and Austrian mother, collapsed. In 1936, when he set out his grand theory of stress, Europe was on the brink of another disastrous conflict, one that would this time subject not just soldiers to the terrible events of conflict but also entire civilian populations, through mass bombing. And, it transpired, when humans are subjected to extreme and sudden stresses which are entirely beyond their control, much like rats, they rapidly become sick.

In September 1940, at the start of the London Blitz, a pair of ingenious medical students, David Winser and D. N. Stewart at the city's Charing Cross hospital, spotted that seven patients had been admitted in a matter of days with perforated stomach ulcers, a serious medical emergency in which the ulcer has made a hole in the digestive tract. Normally their hospital saw about one such case per month. The students wrote to eighteen other London hospitals and asked to view patient records from 1937 to 1940 to understand if there was a wider pattern. Even with some hiccups – one of the hospitals they approached had been bombed out of action – it soon became clear that there was.

The eventual findings, published in the February 1942 edition of medical journal *The Lancet*, showed that in the 'control period' of January 1937 to August 1940, the average total for monthly admissions for perforated ulcers across the sixteen hospitals that returned data was twenty-five. This shot up to an average of sixty-four per month for September and October 1940, when the bombs started falling. After considering various potential reasons, including 'hastily-swallowed meals', or an understandable rise in alcohol and tobacco consumption, the pair concluded: 'The probable cause for this increase was anxiety.'[8]

In 1944, the same duo contributed to a follow-up *Lancet* article showing that over the whole course of the Blitz, from September 1940 to May 1941, the monthly average dipped slightly from the first weeks of the Blitz but at thirty-five remained well above the control period. When the Blitz ended, it fell.[9] This was Selye's alarm stage and resistance stage in action, and even showing one of the same symptoms: stomach ulcers.

Around the same time, the Royal Society of Medicine led an urgent inquiry into the astonishingly high rates of digestive disorders among British troops sent to France with the British Expeditionary Force, or BEF, which ended up being evacuated from Dunkirk in May and June 1940. Statistics showed that nearly 15 per cent of all BEF personnel invalided to the UK before Dunkirk were sent back because of ulcers. However, the report, by two senior doctors, discounted the idea that psychological factors might be involved, instead blaming the excessive eating of over-fatty military food.[10]

Far away from the bombing, in Montreal, Selye was paying attention. In a letter to *The Lancet* in February 1943, he noted the studies about ulcers and the disagreement over the cause. He pointed to the way his stressed rats had also developed ulcers, saying there was increasing evidence for his idea of 'a syndrome which represents the somatic expression of a general alarm of the organism when suddenly presented with a critical situation'[11] – that is to say, chronic stress creates physical consequences.

Selye had been a very busy man. Gathering funding from government agencies and drug companies, among others, he oversaw a huge range of studies. Many were based around artificial steroids, including their potential to dull pain and exhaustion, something of particular interest to the US military, for whom Selye had an additional role as a consultant. Between his arrival at McGill University in 1932 and his departure for Montreal University in 1945, Selye co-authored close to 300 academic papers, as well as writing a four-volume *Encyclopaedia of Endocrinology*. In 1946, Selye published a greatly extended exposition of his general adaptation syndrome, running to over a hundred pages. There was just one problem:

this undoubted productiveness was not reflected in his professional renown. Even Walter Bradford Cannon, the pioneering US physiologist who, just three years before Selye's 1935 breakthrough with rats, devised the concept of homeostasis (about which we will hear a lot more later in the book), was not a fan. Cannon, to whom Selye dedicated his 1946 article, criticized what he said was limited laboratory work to substantiate the theory. Others said that they, too, could not fully trace the path of evidence from injected rats to stressed humans. One argued that Selye's idea was ultimately circular, summarizing it as: 'Stress, in addition to being itself and the result of itself, is also the cause of itself.'[12]

While buffeted and even wounded by the scepticism, Selye was too self-confident to give up or look again at his theories. As one slightly weary book reviewer put it, 'Dr Selye is a man of many things. One of them is not modesty.'[13] Instead, as the 1950s began, he decided to take his ideas to the masses. And this, even more than the scientific papers he produced, really changed how the world saw stress.

The global phenomenon

The process began with lecture tours by Selye across the US and Canada, the talks packaged into a popular 1952 book, *The Story of the Adaptation Syndrome*. By the mid-1950s, Selye's ideas were being quoted in *Healthy Minds and Bodies*, an illustrated guide for British families promising answers to 'all medical, marriage and motherhood problems'. It noted: 'Professor Selye's conclusion to date is that stress is an important factor in the causing of all physical diseases, except, of course, those due to injury, infection or poisoning. This, as you can see, is a very forcible reminder that Worry Can Kill.'[14]

In 1956, Selye produced his own everyday guide to his ideas. *The Stress of Life* became an international bestseller, was translated into more than a dozen languages and still on sale today. Partly a scientific memoir, partly an early self-help guide, Selye began by recounting the progress towards his breakthrough with the help of diagrams and the occasional unsettling photo of a dead laboratory rat. In some ways the message was strikingly modern, particularly the link Selye made between chronic stress and inflammatory ailments including type 2 diabetes. Other parts felt more curious, such as a list for the reader of signs they might be stressed, ranging from the fairly obvious – 'an overwhelming urge to cry, or run and hide' – to the more niche, like high-pitched laughter.[15]

What is striking is how Selye viewed his theory as not just one aspect of health but the key connecting virtually all ailments – as he put it, 'a unified concept of disease'. This was a highly individualistic concept. Each man, Selye wrote – and he was mainly addressing men – has 'an inescapable natural urge to work egotistically for things that can be stored to strengthen his homeostasis in the unpredictable situations with which life may confront him', adding: 'The penalties for failure in this great process of adaptation are disease and unhappiness.'[16]

The alternative idea, that any given man, or woman, might simply be born into inescapable circumstances which might make this head-on confrontation with stress difficult or impossible to win, was not, seemingly, considered. Such an alternative avenue of quieter, less heroic despair was instead becoming the province of pharmaceutical companies. In 1955, a year before *The Stress of Life* was published, Wallace Laboratories launched Miltown, the reassuringly-monikered brand name for meprobamate, the first commercially available tranquillizer in the US. Within two years it accounted for a third of all prescriptions written by American doctors.

Selye was not among the customers. In fact, he seemed almost inexhaustible. Numerous colleagues noted the paradox that the twentieth century's most prominent guru of stress worked between ten and fourteen hours a day, including weekends and holidays, preceded by a pre-dawn swim and a cycle ride to work. As well as his endless stream of articles, books and research papers, he embarked on regular international lecture tours, also managing to fit in three marriages and five children.

As his ideas disseminated through laudatory articles in magazines like *Time* and *Readers' Digest*, Selye also began floating more overtly political notions. In a later book, *Stress Without Distress*, he argued against excessive altruism, saying that people needed an incentive to work. Without this, he warned, a man 'is likely to seek destructive, revolutionary outlets to relieve his basic need for self-assertive activity'.[17]

Selye's ideas began to take on a life of their own. At the start of the 1970s an enterprising New York freelance journalist-turned-self-created-seer called Alvin Toffler released a hugely successful and very obviously Selye-influenced book called *Future Shock*. The title described a phenomenon which Toffler called 'the psychological state that occurs when individuals or societies experience too much change in too little time'.[18] *Future Shock*, which ended up being the first in a best-selling trilogy, tapped into readers' worries and sense of disorientation as the world moved at pace, introducing them to terms like 'information overload'. Two years later, it was made into a documentary presented by Orson Welles. 'We live in an age of anxiety, and a time of stress,' the cigar-puffing director boomed as he was filmed walking through an airport. 'We are the victims of our own technological strength. The victims of shock – of future shock.'[19]

A few years later, Selye and Toffler joined forces to set up the American Institute of Stress, described as 'a clearinghouse for information on all stress-related subjects'.[20] The stated remit might have been broad but the founding board of trustees was illustrative of a slightly more focused view of the phenomenon: alongside various doctors and other experts were a series of Republican politicians, including the party's former presidential candidate, Barry Goldwater, as well as Bob Hope, the entertainer and close friend of Richard Nixon. This was not an organization about to advocate for society-wide reforms to alleviate stress.

Another founder was a US cardiologist, Ray Rosenman, who

was in his own way almost as influential as Selye. Along with a colleague, Meyer Friedman, Rosenman devised the idea of the 'Type A personality', a set of traits which, the pair argued, generated so much pressure and stress, much of it self-imposed, that these people were particularly prone to heart disease.

While getting a heart attack is not notably aspirational, Rosenman and Friedman's portrayal of the Type A personality was. These people were driven, single-minded, competitive, highly ambitious and often successful, cementing the idea of stress predominantly affecting the well-off and busy. They turned the research into a popular 1974 book, *Type A Behavior and Your Heart*, subtitled, *The Cardiologists Who Have Identified the Number One Cause of Heart Attack Give You the Life-saving Facts*.[21]

The idea was not simply made-up. Rosenman and Friedman carried out a series of studies based on long-term surveys covering thousands of men – again, it was just men – which concluded that Type A traits were a predictor of heart disease even when other factors like tobacco use and blood pressure were accounted for. However, subsequent research was unable to replicate the findings. Stress was certainly a factor in heart disease, but it didn't appear to be linked to any particular personality type. It seemed a mystery.

One possible answer, as uncovered decades later through the diligent research of academics such as Mark Petticrew, a British professor of public health, was the influence of the tobacco industry. Using previously confidential documents released by cigarette firms following legal settlements, Petticrew discovered that of the four studies which purported to show a link between Type A traits and heart disease, in three of the cases the researchers either had money from or contact with the tobacco industry.[22]

There was, of course, a very obvious incentive for tobacco firms to portray stress and personality traits as the medical villains. As the evidence mounted up about tobacco's health risks, muddying the waters bought time and put politicians off the regulatory scent. An exaggerated, simplified narrative of stress as inherent and individual served as a particularly good stand-in.

Hans Selye and the tobacco industry

If the development of the Type A personality theory of stress was tainted by cigarette money, the same was true for Hans Selye himself, and arguably more so. Always keen to obtain research money from as many sources as possible, Selye first raised the idea of sponsorship with a tobacco firm in 1958, only to be refused.

But the contacts did not end there. Research into recently released tobacco industry documents shows that throughout the 1960s and 70s, Selye repeatedly received money for projects from major cigarette firms like Philip Morris and discussed with them how his expertise could promote the idea that factors other than tobacco, such as stress, were also a major contributor to illness.

While there is no evidence of a deal, whether formal or implicit, the tobacco firms provided a stream of grants to Selye and his colleagues while he argued against tougher restrictions on smoking. 'The question is not to smoke or not to smoke, but to smoke or drink, eat, drive a car, or simply fret,' Selye told a Canadian parliamentary hearing in 1969 concerning possible tobacco advertising restrictions and health warnings. 'Often more damage is done by creating, through well-meant crusades of enlightenment, innumerable hypochondriacs whose main sickness is really the fear of sickness.'[23]

For years to come, tobacco firms and trade bodies used Selye's arguments to push against health warnings or other curbs in a series of other countries.

A wider perspective

As Selye and his supporters stuck by their almost noble idea of stress as a challenge to be either embraced or fought off, new research was arriving from people with different perspectives.

Cary Cooper is a US-born psychologist who has spent almost

his entire, very long career working in the UK. In 1978 he was one of only two British-based experts asked to join the founding board of the American Institute of Stress. Cooper, who is still heavily involved in the psychology world in his eighties, argues that there was more than just politics or ideology involved when it came to the individualistic approach of Selye and those he gathered around him; it was also the fact that, like Selye, they were almost all doctors.

'The institute was basically the great and the good of American medicine,' Cooper recalls. 'As far as I can remember, I don't think there was another psychologist on the board apart from me. And medics are trained to look at the individual. All those people looking at stress in the US at the time were thinking about was, "How do we treat people who are showing coronary artery disease, how do we reduce their Type A behaviour and prevent them having a heart attack?"

'As a psychologist, my perspective was what the wider environment was doing to damage people's health. Yes, I knew individual differences were important, but that's all the medics would go after, because that's their job.'

The gradual arrival of researchers from other fields helped shift the focus for the study of stress, making it open to a wider range of contributing factors, also encouraging examination of its effects on people other than men in the workplace.

In 1967, a pair of psychiatrists from the University of Washington, Thomas Holmes and Richard Rahe, published what they called the Social Readjustment Rating Scale,[24] usually known as the 'life stress scale'. This was in some ways quite straightforward. It listed forty-three life events and awarded a varying number of points for any that had happened to someone during the past year, ranging from 100 (death of a spouse) to 11 (committing a minor violation like a motoring fine). The scores were totted up, with a total of 300 or more supposedly giving an 80 per cent chance of stress-related illness in the next two years. A total of 150–300 reduced this to 50 per cent, and 150 or less put it below 30 per cent.

There was a method to the idea. Holmes and Rahe first based the list on answers given by 5,000 patients. A study, three years later, of 2,500 US sailors backed up the findings.[25] The idea has obvious limitations and the original 1967 list is hopelessly out of date, with potential stressors including 'Wife beginning or ceasing work outside the home' and 'Taking on a mortgage greater than $10,000.' In adapted forms, the life stress scale is still used, albeit mainly as a self-help guide. It does, however, largely view stress as the result of big, one-off events, not the routine troubles of more everyday life.

It took a group of US psychologists to give an alternative view with a 1981 paper which set out what they called the Hassles and Uplifts Scale.[26] Dispensing with just divorce, death and financial ruin, it asked people to indicate how frequently they had faced one of 117 difficulties, from the big – poor health in a family member – to the more minor, like losing things, having to wait and filling in forms. This was countered with 135 uplifts, ranging from 'knowing your job is safe' and the delightfully-phrased 'becoming pregnant or contributing thereto' to 'daydreaming' and 'flirting'. This wider scale of sometimes more domestically linked woes helped to finally shift the focus beyond the perpetually male stress-world that Selye had set in motion. Unlike the life stress scale, which was tested on sailors, an all-male group, this new scale had more female participants than males. Among the hassles listed were ideas which moved stress beyond the office and into the world that many US women in 1981 were all too familiar with, such as 'preparing meals' and feeling 'overloaded with family responsibilities'.

The research team concluded that for both women and men, 'hassles were a more powerful predictor of psychological symptoms than life events in every comparison made'. Even the scientists involved seemed less likely to be spending their leisure time with Barry Goldwater or Bob Hope than Selye and Toffler. The lead author, Allen Kanner, went on to devise the field of ecopsychology, which connects people to environmentalism. This was beginning to feel like a change of the intellectual guard.

In 1983, eight months after Hans Selye's death, *Time* magazine, which at the time boasted global sales of nearly 6 million copies weekly and a readership of 30 million, featured on its cover a picture of a middle-aged businessman shouting in anguish above the headline '*STRESS! Seeking Cures For Modern Anxieties*'.[27] The article inside included Selye-type orthodoxies and the occasional 'future shock' worry about how to cope with 'everything from the nuclear threat to job insecurity to the near assassination of the President [Ronald Reagan had been shot and wounded two years earlier] to the lacing of medicines with poisons'. But elsewhere within its 5,500-word overview were yet more signs that stress was moving on. Discussing whether major life events or minor troubles were the bigger cause, it quoted not a doctor or even a psychologist but a sociologist, Leonard Pearlin, who argued that both could be true. Using the example of divorce, Pearlin, a pioneer of the sociology of mental illness, said that it 'is not an isolated event – it is accompanied by some social isolation, a reduction in income and sometimes the problems of being a single parent. These become the chronic strains of life.'

The article also pointed to new research highlighting poverty, deprivation and other social factors as likely indicators of stress-related ill health. People living near Los Angeles airport had been found to have a greater chance of developing high blood pressure or heart disease than people in quieter areas, it pointed out. Another recent study had looked at mortality rates across the US state of Massachusetts and identified people living in two so-called death zones, in working-class areas of Boston, as being most at risk. The researcher behind this insight, David Jenkins, was a psychologist who had moved into epidemiology, the science of population-wide health outcomes, again showing how the study of stress was widening its horizons.

Perhaps most notable of all, the article devoted a paragraph to a still little-known study published a year or so earlier in a public health journal. Led by Robert Karasek, a US psychologist who had spent years based in Denmark and Sweden, this used data from a rolling, nationally-run survey of tens of thousands of Swedish workers, comparing heart disease rates with the types of jobs people did. Perhaps not surprisingly, when people described the jobs as 'hectic and psychologically demanding' they seemed more likely to develop heart disease. But there was also another risk factor – what Karasek and his co-authors described as a combination of 'low decision latitude' and limited work-schedule freedom.[28] It was not just being busy that seemed particularly stressful – it was also a lack of control.

This was the beginning of a new way to understand stress – the first openings of a post-Hans-Selye era of viewing it in at least an approximation of the real world. But things were also changing fast in the scientific side of the discipline. Every scientific description of stress, from Selye's general adaptation syndrome onwards, is in essence little more than a way to describe the cumulative impact of those most subtle and mysterious of bodily chemical messengers, our hormones. And it is to these that we turn next.

CHAPTER 3

The Hormones that Shape Your Life

The study of hormones, formally known as endocrinology, is still a relatively new science. The first, very basic experiment into their effects took place as recently as 1848, with the word 'hormone' itself not coined until 1905. And as we shall see in this chapter, while the essence of what hormones do is quite simple to understand, 150 years after that first experiment, there is still a lot we don't know about them.

Hormones, in the simplest definition, are signalling molecules carried around the body via the blood. They only take effect when they bind to specific receptors, which are either on the surface of target cells or within the cells themselves. This interaction triggers cellular responses that, ultimately, lead to physiological changes in the body.

The fifty-plus natural hormones so far identified are produced by the three sections of the endocrine system. First are the glands, for example the pineal and pituitary glands in the brain, the thyroid at the front of the neck and the adrenal glands at the top of the kidneys. Next are the endocrine organs, including the insulin-producing pancreas, the testes and ovaries, and also bodily fat. The latter might sound anomalous, but the role of body fat as an active part of the body's metabolic system, rather than just an inert site for storage, has repercussions for both health and weight, as we will see later on.

The hypothalamus, deep within your brain, performs a crucial organizing role, sending out so-called 'releasing' hormones, which spark other parts of the endocrine system into action, as well as inhibiting hormones, which work the other way round. It also secretes its own hormones. It is variously described as an endocrine gland, an organ, or neither.

Additionally, there are organs which produce hormones but primarily do another job so are not generally treated as full members of the endocrine team, like the liver, heart and digestive tract. More recently, the network of skeletal muscle has been recognized as an endocrine organ. It produces substances called myokines, which while not officially hormones – they are proteins – play a role in key bodily functions like glucose metabolism and bone strength by helping the muscular system communicate with a series of other organs, including the brain, liver and fat tissue. This is fairly new science. The first myokine was identified less than twenty years ago, and researchers are still uncovering the seemingly major influence these proteins have on relieving symptoms of stress, for example by making insulin work more efficiently.

Hormones have a pretty big job: they are in charge of the body's development and growth, as well reproduction, the immune system and the wider metabolism, including everything from the balance of sugars in the blood, our body temperature and heart rate, to things like mood and our sleep cycle. These systems are each maintained by a different set of hormones, all working together at once. In a healthy, well-functioning body they combine in a complex, self-regulating and ever-adjusting mix, one which adapts to both external factors and our inner state. This is a balance very easily knocked off-kilter, whether by ill health, lifestyle factors or, as we have seen with the adrenaline and cortisol-producing adrenal glands, by stress.

As well as being a relatively new science, endocrinology is still only partially understood. The all-pervading and yet subtle work of hormones has, over the decades, proved both tricky to grasp and fertile ground for over-simplistic theories and occasional wild ideas.

Much like stress itself, hormones have, at times, tended to be as much a cultural notion as a purely biological one.

That first properly effective experiment into hormones took place in Germany in August 1848, and given the almost entirely male dominance of science at the time, it's probably not too much of a surprise to learn that the subject chosen for study was the testicles.

Arnold Berthold, a well-travelled German surgeon who had by then settled into life as a lecturer in the university city of Göttingen, took six young cockerels and divided them into three pairs. One pair was castrated, in the next, each bird had a single testicle removed, while the third pair of cockerels were castrated but each then had a testicle from the middle group transplanted into their abdomens.

The results, Berthold reported the following year in the Berlin-based scientific journal known as *Müller's Archive of Anatomy and Physiology*, were striking. The first two birds acted like typical capons, the name for cockerels which are castrated or chemically neutered at a very young age to improve the quality of their flesh. They were 'cowardly in behaviour, were not attracted by the female and exhibited a decidedly capon crow', Berthold reported. The birds with one remaining testicle acted as normal cockerels, he wrote, although when one of them was dissected it was found that its single testicle was notably larger than normal. Most notably, the castrated birds into which a testicle had been implanted seemed no different from any other cockerels, 'showing well-developed wattles, combs and crows, and behaved as males'.

When these birds were dissected, Berthold found the transplanted glands were supplied with new blood vessel connections and appeared to be functioning normally, producing sperm. This showed there was no specific nerve for testicles, meaning what secretions they released internally within the body were passed through the blood, Berthold concluded.

The first public airing of the word 'hormone', in June 1905, took place when the English physiologist Ernest Starling gave a lecture to the Royal College of Physicians in London about endocrinology as it was thus far understood. Hormones were 'chemical messengers', he explained to the audience, which were carried by the bloodstream 'from the organ where they are produced to the organ which they affect'. He devised this new word from *ormao*, the Greek word for 'I excite' or 'I arouse', after consulting William Vesey, a noted classics scholar.

Still under forty, striking in his looks and generally acknowledged as brilliant, if apt to be brusque, Starling was the public face of a scientific double act with another pioneer in the field, the more softly-spoken William Bayliss. The pair were not only long-time collaborators and friends but also brothers-in-law, after Bayliss married Starling's sister, Gertrude. By the time the lecture took place, they had already made their most notable discovery. Inveterate experimenters, in 1902 they carried out an unpleasant-sounding procedure on an anaesthetized dog in which they picked away the nerves around the gut to see if, after this happened, the pancreas would still release digestive juices under stimulus, which it did.[1] This essentially disproved the hypothesis of the even more famous dog-experimenter Ivan Pavlov, who believed the release of digestive juices was controlled by nerves and who won the 1904 Nobel Prize in Physiology for this notion.

To further test their alternative hypothesis that the process involved something secreted into the blood, as Berthold had demonstrated with the testes, Starling and Bayliss took a sample from the dog's intestine after digestion had been simulated and injected it into another dog. That dog's pancreas duly sprung into action. They named the mystery agent 'secretin', which it is still called today. It is generally known as the first hormone to be identified – although, as we shall see in a moment, even this is up for debate.

The hunt for hormones

Secretin is not officially a stress hormone, although, as with much of the endocrine system, it can be affected by stress – one study found that its presence increased between three- and six-fold in the blood of a group of military cadets led on a lengthy march and deprived of sleep. The other hormone which makes the claim to be the first one fully identified and isolated is, in contrast, central to the stress response: adrenaline.

In the 1880s a doctor in Harrogate, Yorkshire, George Oliver, started testing the effects of a series of extracts from animal glands. One much-repeated if never confirmed element of the story is that some of Oliver's experiments were conducted on his own son. After finding that an extract from the adrenal gland appeared to increase blood pressure, he collaborated with the better-resourced and more experienced Edward Schäfer, a professor of physiology at University College London. Using tests on animals rather than family members, the pair showed that the extract did indeed increase blood pressure. Crucially, they also learned that the active substance came from the adrenal medulla, the inner part of the adrenal gland – which, we know now, is the trigger for the fight-or-flight hormonal response.

Their conclusions were published in 1895,[2] and before too long basic adrenal extracts were being used to reduce bleeding in medical procedures. However, they were crude, often causing allergic reactions. The race was on to find the pure substance. This eventually happened in 1901 when adrenaline, the central element in the initial, rapid-reaction part of the stress system, was tracked down by another largely forgotten but fascinating researcher.

Adrenaline

Adrenaline has become the layperson's shorthand for the most basic stress response – most people understand the idea of a rush of adrenaline, causing a fast-pumping heart and heightened attentiveness.

Adrenaline, like noradrenaline, is a type of catecholamine, chemical compounds that provide the first, rapid-reaction part of

> our fight-or-flight stress reaction, as we saw in Chapter 1. As part of the wider HPA axis response, adrenaline, along with noradrenaline, is pumped out by the body in reaction to a shock or threat, instantly increasing blood pressure and pulse, and releasing an instant rush of energy via glucose.

Jokichi Takamine was born in Japan in 1854, just a year after the arrival of US warships had forcibly ended the country's long isolation from the outside world. He trained as a chemist, devising an enzyme that helps break down starch. After relocating to the US, he gave his creation the eponymous brand name of Taka-Diastase and licensed it to a pharmaceutical company as a patented digestive medicine, making him a millionaire. Takamine used his wealth to set up a private laboratory in New York City. With the help of a succession of co-researchers, including the pharmaceutical firm Parke-Davis, he first isolated and then manufactured what he initially called 'glandular extractive product', which was patented under the name 'adrenaline'.

The fact that adrenaline is a trade name has resulted in the slightly confusing situation in which the hormone is known as both adrenaline and epinephrine, its formal scientific moniker. Even more confusingly, while adrenaline was a US patent, the substance tends to be known there as epinephrine, with the UK and much of Europe calling it adrenaline.

Did Takamine beat Starling and Bayliss to the prize of identifying the first hormone? Yes and no. He was first to the post – just, and even though his patented product turned out to also contain noradrenaline (aka norepinephrine), another adrenal-gland hormone which works in a similar way. But others argue that because Takamine isolated the substance from sheep glands rather than observing it in action, the British team deserve the plaudits. Either way, a new period in science had opened – and along with it an entire world of commerce, miracle treatments and, at times, downright quackery.

The Hormone Craze

Adrenaline was soon being used for an array of medical uses, primarily to limit bleeding but also in some therapies which might still be familiar to a modern doctor, such as treating asthma. More ambitious early practitioners claimed it could cure bubonic plague and bedwetting, and if injected at a certain time would allow prospective parents to choose the sex of their child.

As with Arnold Berthold's early work, there was a certain inevitability that, as well as the adrenal glands, the testes would become a major focus. And it was here that things would get a bit curious. In the 1890s a French-US physiologist called Charles-Édouard Brown-Séquard announced that he had injected himself with an extract of testicular fluid taken from guinea pigs and dogs. Despite being well into his seventies, he said he had regained the strength of his youth and, in an eye-opening description at one public lecture, described how he had 'paid a visit' to his much younger wife.[3]

This idea became a lucrative business. In the 1920s, Serge Voronoff, a French surgeon of Russian origin, transplanted parts of the testes of young men who had been executed for serious crimes into the bodies of rich, much older men. This was, very clearly, not a reliable supply so he branched out into using extracts taken from chimpanzees and monkeys. More than 1,000 wealthy men undertook the 'monkey gland treatment', as it was known, with Vonoroff setting up a monkey farm in Italy to meet the demand.

The high point of this rich-men-rejuvenation craze was the work of Eugen Steinach, an Austrian endocrinologist who was simultaneously a genuine pioneer in discovering the functions of sex hormones and, by modern standards, undeniably something of a crank. The first part saw him take forward the unfinished work of Arnold Berthold. Steinach transplanted ovaries into castrated male guinea pigs, and testes into female guinea pigs who had had their sex organs removed, observing how the procedures changed their behaviour. However, unlike Berthold, Steinach did not leave things there. Steinach was a friend of Sigmund Freud and became fascinated with the idea that hormones could also shape less overtly biological characteristics. He decided to take undescended third testes which had been removed from heterosexual men in a routine if rare surgical procedure, and transplant them into gay men. Steinach insisted this then made the men heterosexual.

His most popular invention was something which also had a supposed endocrinological basis. This was the 'Steinach Rejuvenation Procedure', otherwise known as 'being Steinached'. Essentially a part-vasectomy, the twenty-minute mini-operation saw one of a man's two seminal ducts tied off. This was supposed to reinvigorate older men by stimulating the sex glands into a new flurry of activity. In reality, beyond any placebo effect, it did nothing. It didn't even prevent possible pregnancies, as a full vasectomy would have done. Steinach took another view. Setting out his views in a book, *Sex and Life*, he insisted that after the intervention, his patients 'changed from feeble, parched, dribbling drones, to men of vigorous bloom who threw away their glasses, shaved twice a day, dragged loads up to two hundred and twenty pounds, and even indulged in such youthful follies as buying land in Florida.'

However nonsensical this all sounds now, Steinach attracted a string of famous patients and endorsements, among them his friend Freud, who underwent the single snip aged sixty-seven, in 1923. The Irish poet and writer William Butler Yeats was Steinached a decade later, aged sixty-nine, despite worries from his friends that this would be like 'putting a Cadillac engine in a Ford car'. Afterwards, Yeats proclaimed that it had revived his creative powers and granted him a 'second puberty', prompting Irish newspapers to nickname him 'the gland old man'.[4]

Endocrinology was becoming a major business. The Endocrine Society, which remains the largest global organization for the discipline, was formed in New York in 1917 as the Association for the Study of the Internal Secretions. Just seven years later, the brochure for a single US drug company included 116 different remedies based on – or supposedly based on – hormones, including adrenaline for piles and nausea, pituitary-based medicines for constipation, and testicle extracts for epilepsy, cholera, TB and asthma.

There was significant public interest in the idea that hormones could determine all manner of human characteristics, including cognitive behaviour and even personality. This semi-science, known as 'psycho-endocrinology' and also heavily influenced by Freud's writing, was championed by yet another early figure in the field of hormones, who combined very real scientific breakthroughs with some more distinctly off-piste ideas.

Louis Berman was a well-known New York doctor who counted James Joyce and Ezra Pound among his clients. He was a respected endocrine researcher at Columbia University, publishing dozens of papers, and was the first person to isolate the hormone produced by the tiny parathyroid glands in the neck, which regulates the body's calcium levels. Berman was, however, what one historian politely termed 'an audacious extrapolator', with a tendency to take his very real knowledge and run some distance with it. Berman convinced himself that people's individual balance of hormones shaped their characters. In a series of best-selling books he set out what he termed, evocatively if with descriptive licence, 'the chemistry of the soul'. People were, he argued, one of a series of types, depending on which gland was dominant.

As well as surmising, troublingly, that major endocrine differences existed across ethnic groups, Berman believed people's 'glandular make-up' could be gauged from their faces. After spending time studying criminals in New York's Sing Sing prison, Berman argued that much of criminality was a matter of hormonal balance. Murderers, he believed, had too many secretions from the adrenal gland and from the thymus gland, which we now know plays an important role in our immune system. Muggers, in contrast, were low on sex hormones.

As hinted at by the title of his 1938 book *New Creations in Human Beings*, Berman started moving his ideas further and further in the direction of eugenics. If hormones shape who we are, he wrote, they could be changed: 'We will be able to govern man's capacities in every detail so that we can create the ideal human being. The only problem will be the selection of the ideal type.'[5]

The trial of the century

Even today, the bare facts can shock. In May 1924 two rich, privileged and hugely intelligent Chicago students, Nathan Leopold and Richard Loeb, kidnapped a boy, fourteen-year-old Bobby Franks, largely at random. They beat him to death and hid his naked body under a remote embankment outside the city before contacting the boy's wealthy father to pretend he had been kidnapped. And why? Seemingly to show they could get away with it – to commit the perfect crime.

They did not succeed. A pair of spectacles was found near Frank's body, a type stocked by just one Chicago optician, which had sold precisely three pairs – one to Leopold. After the duo were arrested, eventually confessing guilt, the US public became fascinated by the youth, arrogance and distinctive personalities of the killers.

Leopold, known as 'Babe', was the older, at nineteen, and reportedly had an IQ so high it went beyond the scale of measurement. He was, however, socially awkward, unlike his childhood friend Loeb, aka Dickie, who was eighteen at the time of the murder, almost as intelligent, but also notably good-looking and charming. Their crime was the inspiration for the play *Rope*, later made into a film by Alfred Hitchcock.

The killers' wealthy parents hired not only the most celebrated defence lawyer of the period, Clarence Darrow, but a series of medical experts to examine Leopold and Loeb in prison. The plan was for them to plead guilty to the killing but claim their mental conditions meant they were not responsible. And in a direct echo of Louis Berman's ideas, a key part of this defence was glands.

> A medical report submitted to the trial said both suffered differing forms of glandular disorders. Loeb had 'multi-gland dysfunction', while Leopold had malfunctions of the pituitary and pineal glands. Newspapers were provided with profile pictures of the pair featuring arrows pointing to various glands and their associated personality traits, such as 'Destructive Instinct' and 'Love of Excitement'.
>
> The judge, John R. Caverly, said that while he accepted such studies had relevance to crimes in general, he discounted the defence and found the pair guilty of murder. They escaped the death penalty only because of their youth.

The search for cortisol

Away from the noise of psycho-endocrinology and men hawking testicular extracts, others were getting on with hormonal breakthroughs which would prove vastly more significant, particularly connected to the hormone which is at the centre of our story – cortisol.

One US chemist, called Edward Kendall, was so committed to his mission to isolate and utilize new bodily secretions that his autobiography would be subtitled *Memoirs of a Hormone Hunter*.[6] In 1914, Kendall became the first scientist to isolate thyroxine, the primary hormone secreted by the thyroid gland, which has a wide-ranging role in metabolism, heart and muscle function. He then set to work on the adrenal system, a task that would occupy him for more than two decades.

By the mid-1930s Kendall and his co-researchers at the Mayo Clinic, Minnesota, had used cow adrenal glands to isolate a series of as-yet unnamed hormones, labelled only as compounds A to F. Gradually, their structure was unpicked, and cortisol, at last, came into proper view: it was compound F. Compound E was cortisone, a biologically inactive variant of cortisol which has become the basis for vast numbers of subsequent drugs and treatments. A and B were also types of cortisol. The isolation of a new adrenal hormone was hugely exciting, especially given all the uses already found for adrenaline. There was just one problem: how to produce any?

Getting even tiny amounts of hormones was, at the time, often a hugely complex and expensive business. In his earlier work, with thyroxine, Kendall had used almost three tonnes of pig thyroid glands to eventually isolate and then crystallize the substance. He then spent a decade trying and failing to determine thyroxine's structure, in part so it could be produced artificially. In the end a British researcher beat him to it.

To finance his subsequent work, Kendall extracted adrenaline on behalf of a pharmaceutical company in return for the large stocks of bovine adrenal glands they sent him for free, which he and his team could then use for their own research.

With the advent of the Second World War, the race to produce synthetic adrenal hormones gained new impetus amid rumours that Nazi scientists had managed to produce an extract which allowed German pilots to fly at great altitude without needing additional oxygen. It was, the story went, produced from cattle glands sent to Germany from Argentina. This worry became a near-panic in 1941 when a German submarine was captured travelling back from Argentina carrying a huge cargo of an unidentified meaty mass. While initially assumed to be adrenal glands, this turned out to be liver, and after the war it transpired that the adrenal extract rumour was just that – a rumour.

Nonetheless, the years of effort finally paid off. In 1948 Kendall was able to produce cortisol on a mass scale. His Mayo Clinic colleague Philip Hench persuaded him to use some of the new-supply cortisone, aka compound E, for clinical trials on arthritis. It had notable success in reducing inflammation. A new era of medication had arrived. Kendall and Hench were awarded a share of the 1950 Nobel Prize in Physiology.

After cortisol was isolated, researchers started to fill in the blanks about conditions which had already been identified but were up to that point mysterious. Back in the mid-1850s an English physician called Thomas Addison had identified an ailment in which patients lacked energy and strength, and lost weight. This turned out to be a rare disorder of the adrenal glands in which they do not produce cortisol. Addison's disease, as it is known, was one of the first conditions treated with the hormone.

On the other side of the balance, in 1912 a US doctor called Harvey Cushing had noted something he called 'polyglandular syndrome', with symptoms which also included weakness, as well as a build-up of fat around the stomach and on the neck, and a puffy face.[7] Cushing's syndrome, it turned out, was usually caused by a benign tumour in the pituitary gland. The result? More cortisol than the body can handle. Once again, when it comes to hormones, it is all about the correct balance.

Ninety or so years since cortisol was isolated, what do we know about it? The brief answer is: a lot, and yet by no means everything.

Cortisol output is controlled, as we have already heard, by the HPA axis, connecting the brain with the pituitary gland and is central to our body's stress response. Cortisol is pumped into the body in two conjoined patterns. The first is a broad twenty-four-hour process in which concentrations peak in the morning, as we wake, and gradually decrease towards the late evening, a timing led by the suprachiasmatic nucleus, a central bodily clock within the hypothalamus. Within this wider curve is what is called an ultradian pattern, in which pulses of cortisol are released at various points. And finally, of course, it is released under stress, whether sudden or chronic.

The non-stressed daily rhythm seems relatively fixed. Experiments in which scientists mimicked night-shift work, by having subjects stay awake at night and sleep during the day, slightly delayed when the peak of cortisol was emitted, but there was no apparent wider change in either the overall volume or the pattern.

What does appear to upset things is flux. A frankly sadistic-sounding experiment saw a group of young men – who, we are assured, volunteered for the task – spend three weeks living under what was effectively a 24.6-hour clock: each day, the laboratory lights which designated the start and end of the eight-hour sleep period were turned off and then on again thirty-six minutes later. At the end of this process, average cortisol levels had dropped significantly.[8]

More widely, consistently poor sleep is known to be both a cause of stress and a common symptom of it. Separate experiments have seemed to show that extended periods of sleep deprivation can cause cortisol levels to rise, although the results have been mixed. But what is clear is sleep deprivation is linked to insulin resistance. One study found a notable rise in both insulin levels and insulin resistance among women of varying ages when their sleep time was shortened.[9]

Circadian or diurnal?

There are four types of biological rhythm in the human body, and two are very easy to understand. Ultradian ones are shorter than a day, like the way cortisol is released in pulses. Infradian are longer than a day, for example the menstrual cycle. The other two, circadian and diurnal, can seem similar, and the ebb and flow of cortisol tends to be described as both interchangeably. Circadian simply means over a 24-hour cycle, irrespective of external factors, while diurnal implies some sort of synchronization with day and night, or light and dark.

So which does cortisol actually follow? Both, really. There is a day/night element in the way it peaks in the blood around the time people wake up and then gradually declines towards evening. But some scientists argue it is circadian as there is a full 24-hour cycle, including how it builds up in the night before people wake. So take your pick.

When it comes to the cognitive impact of cortisol, the picture is nuanced. One thing is certain: cortisol is a very brain-centred hormone. Aside from being triggered by the HPA axis, the brain is full of so-called binding sites for corticoids, the group of hormones including cortisol. These binding sites come in two types, mineralocorticoid receptors and glucocorticoid receptors. These are slightly different in function. Mineralocorticoid receptors are what's known as high-affinity receptors, slightly more sensitive to cortisol, and they function all the time, even when levels are minimal. In contrast, glucocorticoid receptors are low-affinity and generally kick in either during the natural daily peak, or when there is a stress-related rush.

One particularly notable fact is that these receptors, when triggered by cortisol, act as something known as a transcription factor. Transcription factors are bodily proteins which, in a very simplified sense, interpret messages on behalf of the cells that are affected by them. These play a role in more or less every aspect of human biology, even down to determining our sex. Recent research has shown that the way transcription factors operate can be changed by stress.

All this may sound complicated, but it translates into a very crucial point: to once again simplify things somewhat, the action of cortisol on our body is not a direct, predictable, constant process. It is, in effect, something interpreted by the brain. This is yet another reason why people can react to cortisol in very different ways.

Both types of receptors are particularly abundant in the hippocampus, the part of the brain central to learning and memory, and in the medial prefrontal cortex, which is connected to a range of functions including decision-making, long-term memory and emotion.

The impact of cortisol on memory is yet another example of its sometimes contradictory effects. As we saw in Chapter 1, long-term stress can make it harder for people to focus on things beyond immediate problems and can even dull their general cognitive function. But shorter bursts of cortisol can actually improve people's memories – at least in part.

Tests on students about to take exams, who had higher-than-usual levels of both perceived stress and of cortisol, showed that they performed notably better in a simple word-recall test than they did during a more relaxed, non-exam period, when their cortisol was lower. But when asked to do more complex tasks, for example counting up a tally of recorded bleeps while simultaneously searching in a phone directory, they performed notably worse while stressed.[10]

Other experiments have indicated that although increased cortisol can boost short-term memory, it tends to make people less good at converting these into longer-term recollections, a process associated with the hippocampus, which is particularly well-stocked with glucocorticosteroid receptors.

This returns us to a familiar point: much as stress is inescapable, it is not always a bad thing. Elevated cortisol can have its uses. It is all about the extent, and in some cases the individual. One German study tried to work out whether stress might help people perform better in a competitive environment. Given that it is hard to take cortisol swabs during physical sport, they used a video-game tournament. The researchers found that the players who showed barely any increase in cortisol levels from their base levels did the worst. Those with the highest change in cortisol performed moderately. It was the players who had some extra cortisol, but not too much, who won the most games.[11]

Predictability and stress

As we have already seen, the problems come when the HPA axis is repeatedly and chronically triggered. We look at the wider biological mechanisms of this in the next chapter. But when it comes to cortisol and the general fight-or-flight hormonal response, there are some useful basics to know.

We have seen how control, or even a perception of control, is an important element in managing the impacts of stress. Another one, known about for decades, is the idea of predictability. If you recall the study in Chapter 2 about the surge in stomach ulcers during the London Blitz, some modern retellings of the research add an intriguing detail. While the stress-related increase in perforated ulcers was witnessed across the capital, they say, it was more pronounced in the outer suburbs, which unlike the inner city were bombed only occasionally, rather than every night. Although these suburb-dwellers were in much less danger overall, they faced the extra stress of never knowing when the terror would arrive. This is a fascinating finding, but sadly it doesn't feature anywhere in the published research. There is no evidence that the medical students who carried out the study even compared the incidence of ulcers between various parts of the capital.

You can nonetheless see how the myth perpetuated, given that it ties in with what has been shown in subsequent research. In 1970, the US psychologist Jay Weiss carried out yet another of his trade's unpleasant animal experiments, one which demonstrated precisely the link claimed in the imaginary Blitz analysis.

A series of rats were placed inside a restrictive cage mechanism that allowed them to move forwards and backwards but not turn around, and had an electrode attached to their tail. In one group each rat received a mild electric shock exactly ten seconds after a beep was sounded. The other group received the same shocks and also heard a beep, but there was no correlation between the timing of the sound and when the shock was delivered. All the rats were then killed and dissected, and it was found that the animals given the unpredictable shocks showed much greater signs of stomach ulcers.

A follow-up study measured cortisol levels. The rats given no warning of the shocks had much higher concentrations in their blood. They also showed other signs of stress, such as weight loss and going off their food. Further tests demonstrated the same effect irrespective of whether the warning was a noise or a blinking light, or if the rats were restrained or free to move. Predictability was the key.[12]

Another long-known factor in mitigating stress is habituation –

that is to say, getting used to something. This has been shown in all sorts of ways over the years, perhaps most memorably by getting novices to do a series of parachute jumps and measuring their cortisol levels. One example saw staff and students at a German university take a three-jump parachute training course. As you might expect, their cortisol levels, measured every twenty minutes throughout the day, spiked hugely just before the jumps, and on their first jump averaged about nine times the so-called basal concentration, or what you would expect in someone not undergoing stress. These were slightly lower with the second jump and notably so for the third, albeit still well beyond normal levels. Intriguingly, while this was the average trend, some participants did not see their cortisol peaks drop with later jumps.[13] Not everyone becomes used to stressful events, it appears.

Both these ideas make sense in an everyday world beyond rats in cages and students strapped into parachutes. Imagine a dysfunctional workplace with a grumpy, even borderline-abusive boss. While that is very obviously a bad starting point and a very likely prompt for stress, if you went to the office every day knowing you would be shouted at, that might seem easier to prepare for than a boss who bottled up their aggression and flew into a rage at random moments, days or weeks apart. Similarly, the first time the shouting erupted, it would be a shock; by day five, or week two, you would be more used to it. It would still be stressful, not to mention completely unacceptable. But the degree of strain would differ.

To continue the example of the dysfunctional office, another factor that would seem likely to at least partly reduce the overall stress would be supportive colleagues, ones who told you to ignore the boss and that you were good at your job. This can be a surprisingly powerful thing. Much as identity salience, a slightly technical term for the centrality of how we see ourselves, can make people believe damaging stereotypes about themselves, positive reinforcement can do the opposite. Strange as it might sound, people can sometimes cope better with stress just by believing that they can. A striking illustration of this saw a group of university students put through an artificial stress situation which is a staple of such projects. Known as the Trier Social Stress Test, named after the German university where it was devised, even describing how it works is enough to raise a cold sweat.

The standard version involves giving participants a pen and paper and telling them to prepare for a hypothetical job interview. The pen and paper are then unexpectedly taken away early, before they have to give a five-minute presentation to researchers posing as interviewers, who remain silent and expressionless. The 'interviewers' only speak if the participant finishes before the five minutes are up, telling them to carry on. As if that isn't enough, the volunteers are then ordered to spend five more minutes counting backwards from 1,022 in units of thirteen, having to return to the beginning if they make a mistake.

This study added a tweak, however: two days before the stress test, each volunteer filled out an online questionnaire about their ability to cope with stress. The answers they gave were entirely irrelevant – the questionnaire was a red herring. Each student was randomly assigned to one of two groups. After arriving at the laboratory, people in the so-called high-expectancy group were told they had scored very well in this bogus online test and were the type of person likely to cope well with stressful situations. Those in the low-expectancy group were told the opposite – they were the sort who tend to fare badly. Even after accounting for other factors, such as socioeconomic status and personality type, the people who were told they were likely to feel stress showed notably higher cortisol readings than those who were told they would not.[14]

Cortisol is a fascinating marker for stress. But measuring just as a single hormone can give us only one part of the bodily picture. The important thing is how they work together. And it is to this that we look next.

CHAPTER 4

The Need for Homeostasis

Hannah decided to come to Richard's clinic, she said, not for one particular reason but because – and these were almost her very first words – 'Things just don't feel right.'

A lawyer in her early thirties with, as she described it, a happy and fulfilled personal life and a stable family background, Hannah said there were aspects of her health that she simply didn't understand. For one thing, she felt run down a lot of the time, even when she had slept enough. Another mystery, Hannah continued, was that she exercised vigorously and often, sometimes taking three high-intensity gym classes in a week, and also ate well, but never seemed to lose the weight she wanted to. She was doing all the right things, but it wasn't paying off. What was going on?

There was an immediate answer, albeit one that opened up a series of other questions. A blood test showed Hannah had hyperinsulinemia, meaning a higher level of insulin in her blood than would be normal. This was only slight; she was not about to be diagnosed with type 2 diabetes. But it was an indication she could become prediabetic, the precursor to the full condition, with all the potential health issues this entails. Hannah's response was, not unexpectedly, shock. How, she asked, could someone like her end up like this?

How indeed? The answer is a complex one. So far we have described stress and hormones almost as a series of parallel processes and effects. To explain Hannah's story we need to put them all together.

It begins with a would be-playwright who became a doctor almost by chance, and ended up pioneering the way we think about the human body as a cohesive, interconnected whole. Born in 1813 in the Rhône region of south-eastern France, Claude Bernard was the son of a debt-ridden winemaker. His Jesuit schooling involved no science at all, and even when apprenticed to an apothecary, a pharmacy of that era, Bernard spent most of his time writing plays. Such was Bernard's passion for the theatre that in 1834, aged twenty-one, he set out for Paris with a completed five-act tragedy – but was persuaded by a sympathetic literary critic that medicine might me a better use for his talents.

Bernard was at first a mediocre medical student, but gradually proved himself a natural innovator and experimenter, eventually becoming one of the most influential physiologists of the modern age. Earlier discoveries, including the roles of the pancreas and liver in digestion and breaking down fats, led eventually to Bernard's lasting contribution to science, fully set out his 1878 paper *Leçons sur les phénomènes de la vie communs aux animaux et aux végétaux*, or 'Lectures on the phenomena of life common to animals and plants.'[1]

This was a concept he called the *milieu intérieur*, the idea that our body's cells are nourished and maintained within an internal environment that keeps itself in equilibrium, making adjustments as needed depending on external factors.

Bernard's theory, with the idea of an 'internal ocean' bathing the cells, did to an extent mirror the ancient and long-discredited medical notion of 'bodily humors', vital fluids which supposedly govern health. However, his observation about how the body regulated its heat and maintained glucose levels directly paved the way to another concept, one still central to understanding how human bodies function.

This was homeostasis, the brainchild of Walter Bradford Cannon, the US physiologist we encountered briefly in Chapter 2, whose career was notably less chequered than that of Bernard. After choosing to study medicine at Harvard, Cannon settled down and spent his whole career there. His big idea, fully set out in his 1932 book *The Wisdom of the Body*, drew on what was by then more than three decades of Cannon's own research.[2] Unlike the *milieu intérieur*, it remains a vital part of physiological thinking to this day.

In its most basic sense, homeostasis describes the various ways in which the body maintains equilibrium, keeping a balance of variables including core temperature and the levels of glucose and oxygen in the tissues and blood. There are officially two types of homeostasis: predictive and reactive. The first is simply where hormones respond to seasonal or day/night variables, for example how cortisol levels increase naturally just before we wake up.

Reactive homeostasis involves what is known as negative feedback: sensors detect when one of the variables is out of alignment and take action to compensate. Much as a central-heating thermostat would respond to an open window in winter by firing up the boiler, a dropping bodily core temperature prompts shivering and also cutaneous vasoconstriction, the process where blood is directed towards internal organs.

If body-temperature maintenance is one of the more straightforward parts of reactive homeostasis, relatively speaking, then maintaining stable glucose levels is notably more complex. For homeostasis to be in place, blood glucose levels should remain within a very narrow range of 3.9–5.6 millimoles per litre. A millimole, otherwise known as one thousandth of a mole, is a technical unit to express the concentration of something, and is hard to translate into more everyday terms. But it is fair to say that this is not a large amount. This bodily balancing act is carried out by the opposing actions of glucagon and insulin, hormones both produced in the pancreas. Glucagon stimulates glucose production in the liver, increasing your blood sugar levels; insulin does the opposite.

Insulin

What is insulin? In one sense, just one among dozens of hormones. But it is among the most vital and valuable substances in our body – and the source of numerous and alarmingly common ailments and disorders.

Its function is simple but essential. Insulin regulates the concentration of sugars in the blood by helping these enter the body's cells, whether for immediate energy use or storage. In a healthy body, your pancreas is constantly producing the correct amount of insulin to maintain your blood glucose within a healthy range.

The fact that insulin is so vital to our well-being is shown by type 1 diabetes, an autoimmune condition in which the pancreas produces little or no insulin. As we shall see in Chapter 7, before scientists managed to isolate and artificially produce insulin, the life of someone with type 1 diabetes was almost universally difficult and brief.

A much more common ailment is insulin resistance, where the body fails to respond properly to insulin and so it increases how much it secretes. This state of elevated insulin, formally known as hyperinsulinemia, is the pathway to type 2 diabetes, the generally lifestyle-related form of the disease.

When written down, this sounds relatively uncomplicated. But it is not, as demonstrated by estimates suggesting more than a third of all British adults fail to properly maintain blood glucose homeostasis and are thus either prediabetic or already have type 2 diabetes.[3]

Unlike type 1 diabetes, which is an auto-immune condition where the pancreas simply does not make sufficient insulin, its type 2 cousin and the prediabetic state are seen as an ailment of lifestyle, albeit with some help from genetics. Much of it, as we'll detail later in the book, is down to factors like diet, obesity and long-term physical activity. The actual science around precisely how sedentary lifestyles or greater amounts of body fat cause increased insulin resistance is a bit complicated. However, the consensus that it happens is unargued.

This takes us back to the paradox of Hannah, with her regular exercise classes and diet of freshly cooked meals. Her physical regime would seem the antithesis of hyperinsulinemia. To reiterate her own question: what was going on? This brings us to the next stage of our story, and the other major factor in blood glucose homeostasis, which is, as you might have already guessed, stress. And that in turn takes us back to the life and work of Walter Bradford Cannon.

It is probably unfair to contrast Claude Bernard's eventful career with Cannon's lifelong loyalty to Harvard, given that the latter was not spent entirely in the classroom and laboratory. During World War One, Cannon volunteered with the US Army Expeditionary Force, travelling to France where he treated injured soldiers, sometimes under enemy fire, also carrying out experiments into the physiological impacts of shock. He did this despite being in his mid-forties, with a wife and five children at home.

This visceral mid-life experience helped Cannon make two significant advances in understanding how shock affects the body. The first was devising ways to mitigate so-called secondary shock, when a patient's blood pressure and body temperature can plummet. His research noted the vital importance of immediate hydration and warmth, which are still fundamentals of first aid today.

The other legacy of Cannon's stint at the battlefield casualty stations was to advance investigations he had already been making into the significant impact of non-bodily trauma and stress. In 1915, before he went to war, Cannon published a book with the lengthy if eloquent title *Bodily Changes in Pain, Hunger, Fear, and Rage: An Account of Recent Researches into the Function of Emotional Excitement*, which set out, among other things, how emotional triggers alone can prompt the adrenal gland to produce stimulant hormones like adrenaline, a pioneering idea for the time.[4]

While the research behind Cannon's 1915 work was primarily the result of stimulus-and-response experiments using a succession of unfortunate laboratory cats, he was clear about the repercussions for humans and also the way that this stress-created adrenal overload could, in the longer term, affect the delicate balance of blood sugar. Among the examples he cited was a German officer whose experiences in the short but brutal Franco-Prussian war of 1870–71 brought him not just a medal for valour, but subsequent diabetes; and a man who developed the same condition shortly after discovering his wife was having an affair.

Nearly twenty years later, in *The Wisdom of the Body*, Cannon introduced not just one pivotal new idea, homeostasis, but a second: 'fight or flight'.[5] As we have seen, while this ancient hormonal response is common to all vertebrates, humans alone face the very recent (in evolutionary terms) twist of chronic stress repeatedly firing up the second part of this process, the HPA axis. This stress response is very much a brain-led operation, something that was not always understood. Early researchers tended to treat human glands as cooperative but ultimately independent states which released their hormones to maintain balance in their particular area of the body. By the 1930s one pioneering British endocrinologist, Walter Langdon-Brown, got slightly closer by declaring the pituitary gland at the base of the brain to be the 'leader of the endocrine orchestra'.[6]

The truth lay slightly higher up. In the 1940s another British researcher, Geoffrey Harris, who kept a portrait of Claude Bernard above his desk, used experiments on rabbits to show that hormonal responses could be triggered by electrical stimulation directly in the hypothalamus, indicating that it contained some kind of control mechanism. Subsequent research uncovered multiple hypothalamic hormones, many of which are used to nudge other bodily glands into action.

The great rivalry

Two of the scientists who did the most to build on Geoffrey Harris's work in identifying the various secretions produced by the hypothalamus were Roger Guillemin and Andrew Schally. They are known for two things: being innovative and distinguished researchers, and for waging one of science's most famous, bitter and arguably petty, soap-opera-style rivalries.

Guillemin was born in France, interrupting his medical studies to help the French Resistance transfer escaped prisoners across the mountains to Switzerland. After finishing his training, he relocated to Canada, working with Hans Selye, before settling in America. Schally, born Andrzej Schally in Poland, fled the Nazi invasion in 1939, first to Romania and then the UK, also eventually living in America, after a period in Canada.

Given that they both ended up in the same country after such similar trajectories, and worked in the same field of research, you might expect the duo to have collaborated. And this did happen – Schally briefly worked in Guillemin's laboratory. However, the research faltered and they both blamed each other.

This began a hugely rancorous two-decade race to be first in isolating the same hypothalamic hormones. Often, scientists in the same field willingly swap ideas. Schally and Guillemin, whose rivalry was often caricatured as the personality differences of a blunt Slav versus a more urbane Frenchman, instead set up rival teams of researchers to do precisely the same work. Guillemin even declined to credit Schally's studies in his own papers.

It was Schally who won the race, by a whisker, in identifying the initial substance, known as thyrotropin-releasing hormone – his paper on the subject was published just six days before that of Guillemin. The US-Pole also narrowly won with the second secretion, hormone-releasing hormone, but Guillemin triumphed with the third, somatostatin.

> The Nobel academy tried to end the argument by jointly awarding them a share of the 1977 Prize in Physiology or Medicine, but their rivalry continued, later chronicled in a best-selling book, *The Nobel Duel*.[7]

What does all this mean for Hannah? It means that if some of her health concerns did have a basis in excessive cortisol levels, which seemed likely, then it would not be an entirely straightforward fix. This stress response is not simply a matter of physiology, but also psychology and environment. Beyond things like exercise and diet, she needed to consider her home and work, her childhood, even her gender.

Fight-or-flight and the subsequent role of the HPA axis can sound, when described, an almost mechanistic process. But it is never the same in any two people, even down to the way the same amount of cortisol can affect different people, which can be in extremely different ways – very often a product of people's backgrounds and infancy.

Numerous studies have shown that a mother's exposure to consistently high cortisol during pregnancy tends to make their child less able to deal with the physiological manifestations of stress when they are an adult. Arguably most crucial is the early environment for babies, who take several months to build a circadian rhythm for cortisol and which is not fully in place until they are aged around four. This is, of course, almost always due to circumstances beyond the mother's control. But while it should not be a reason for shame or stigma, it is a biological fact.

We discuss the central role of the early years of life more fully in Chapter 9, but to understand homeostasis and the way it can be knocked off-course, we need to outline the basics. To put it simply: babies are not designed to deal with stress on their own. Their brains require their needs to be met, which involves not just the necessity of feeding, but touch, holding, stimulation and attention. Babies denied this can see naturally low cortisol levels soar, something which can affect the development of neurotransmitter systems. Such babies tend to grow up with fewer cortisol receptors in the hippocampus, making them less able to deal with a stress-released flood of cortisol.

One Canadian study took a group of young people and assessed their family backgrounds and parental relationships before sending them out with a diary to record stressful experiences, as well as a series of saliva swabs to measure their cortisol four times a day. The researchers' conclusion was blunt: 'The less parental warmth individuals received during childhood, the more cortisol they secreted on days that they experienced more severe stress.'[8]

Some of the start-of-life triggers for this tendency are perhaps as you might expect, for example parental addiction or extreme family turmoil. Others, however, shift into more societally contested ground. One of the most controversial areas is research showing that infants, and even younger children, can experience elevated cortisol if regularly separated from their primary caregiver. A landmark study by Andrea Dettling, a German researcher, tested cortisol in preschool children attending a nursery and found high levels even in the afternoon, where under normal circumstances it would be undergoing the gradual wind-down towards the night. The younger the child and the less developed their social skills, the greater this effect.[9]

Research like this can be extremely difficult to digest for many parents who, for a series of often pressing reasons, need to return to work, not least in places like the United States, where statutory maternity leave lasts precisely twelve weeks. However, subsequent studies, some also carried out by Dettling, discovered that, when separated from their parents, if a young child has an easily definable and constant person to attach to, whether a childminder or a relative, the effect disappears. This is not a magic solution, given that nurseries tend to be cheaper and more flexible than childminders, but it can offer some options.

All this takes us back, at last, to Hannah, and the beginnings of an explanation for her health woes. She arrived at the clinic as someone professedly stable and from a family almost boring in its everyday contentment. And it is undeniable that many things had gone well in her early life: a childhood spent not only in the same town but the same house, with parents in professional careers and a younger brother to whom she remains close. But more questioning brought up some potentially significant details.

*

When she was born, Hannah's parents had only recently moved into their home and were struggling to pay the mortgage, making both of them distracted and, in the case of her mother, under pressure to get back to work. Within three months, her mother had done precisely this, leaving Hannah in the care of a grandmother, who then herself became seriously ill, with a local childminder stepping in until Hannah was old enough to attend a local nursery. Her mother later experienced depression, severely so after the birth of Hannah's brother. While, yet again, none of this is the fault of Hannah's parents, let alone of Hannah herself, all this is not, as a psychotherapist might put it, an infancy destined to create a securely attached adult – or, as a stress expert might add, one with a stable and routinely time-driven flow of cortisol.

A few weeks after her blood sugar levels were tested, Hannah took a saliva swab shortly after she woke up to measure her cortisol levels at their morning peak, officially known as the cortisol awakening response. It was higher than ideal, albeit not dramatically so. One-off tests present just a snapshot and a whole-day chart would give a better picture of how stress is manifested. However, research suggests that a high cortisol awakening response is a particular indicator of chronic stress. We were inching closer to an answer.

Further questioning gave signs that Hannah struggled to regulate stress, for example waking up in the middle of the night to worry about a work task she had forgotten, and finding it hard to share her worries with her partner.

Studies have shown that sustained high cortisol can have a variety of damaging effects in the long term – everything from a diminished immune system to impaired memory and a greater propensity to dementia in later life.[10] But what about malfunctioning blood glucose, and – Hannah's complaints on arrival – a tendency to feel worn down and to gain weight? After our diversion into the neurological and psychological backdrop to cortisol, it is time to delve back into the mechanics of physiology.

A body off-balance

How do we know that long-term excess cortisol plays havoc with that delicate homeostatic balance of blood sugars? One very obvious answer comes from observing the symptoms of people who suffer from Cushing's syndrome, as seen in Chapter 3, where people are exposed to excessive cortisol over a prolonged period, sometimes due to a benign tumour in the pituitary gland. One of the defining characteristics of Cushing's syndrome is abnormally high blood sugar levels, along with a series of other effects including weight gain in the abdomen, face and trunk, as well as muscular weakness.

There is also plenty of laboratory evidence about the link between high cortisol and blood sugar. In one particularly straightforward study, groups of volunteers were either infused with a cortisol solution or neutral saline. Those in the former group were then found to have generated more blood glucose and also responded less well to small amounts of insulin.[11]

Hannah does not have Cushing's syndrome, and no one has dosed her artificially with cortisol. But based on her symptoms, and her self-described background, it's a decent bet that her levels of the hormone tend to be high across much of the twenty-four-hour cortisol cycle. This would be likely to explain her high blood insulin reading. So how, in physiological terms, does the first cause the second?

As we saw earlier, when a mass of cortisol circulates the body in response to a perceived threat, following the faster-acting adrenaline, it prompts an upsurge in the release of energy in the form of glucose. Because this is a crisis response, it taps into what you might call the body's short-term-storage energy system. This is glycogen, found in the liver, as opposed to energy stored as triglycerides, a type of fat. Cortisol, however, mainly uses the energy stored in the liver, inhibiting glucose uptake from muscle.

This is a key factor. Skeletal muscle, which constitutes a third or more of the average body mass, plays a vital role in what is formally known as glucose clearance – removing it from the blood for storage, especially after a meal. It can be responsible for 80 per cent or more of this process. To move briefly into even greater specifics, glucose clearance in fat tissues and skeletal muscle is primarily led by something called glucose transporter type 4, which has the evocative acronym of GLUT-4. It is a process stimulated by insulin, and the presence of cortisol makes the insulin less effective. Cortisol also limits the production and secretion of insulin by the pancreas, further raising blood glucose levels.

All this is fine as a one-off, or even an irregular occurrence. Just like the mass-release of adrenaline, the triggering of the HPA and the subsequent flood of longer-lasting cortisol is very much there for an evolutionary reason, and the body can cope with it. But for someone like Hannah, with an infancy that primed her for cortisol release under stress, coupled with a modern lifestyle that makes such stress all but unavoidable, her metabolic alarm system is triggered on a routine and chronic basis. The hormonal 'brake' of the parasympathetic nervous system, intended to wind back the hormonal response, as we saw in the first chapter, is not then able to calm things down. And that is when the problems begin to mount up.

One of the fundamentals of homeostasis is that when things go wrong, the body's attempts to restore balance can end up becoming not a one-off process of correction but a damaging feedback loop. Thus, if insulin is working less well, then the pancreas tries to put this right by producing more of it to try to maintain blood sugar levels. This is known as hyperinsulinemia. And if it gets to a point where the pancreas can no longer produce enough insulin to process the endless cortisol-prompted blood sugars, then this can be a pathway towards diabetes. The constant cortisol has upset the balance. To resurrect the home-heating parallel from earlier in the chapter, rather than the idea of having a boiler fire up to compensate for an open window, this is like having both the heating and air conditioning on at the same time, battling each other before eventually one or both stop working.

Such a situation, in physiological terms, is the opposite of homeostasis, and it has its own antonym: allostasis. This is a body out of kilter, going beyond its limits, no longer seeking equilibrium. In the natural world, allostasis can at times be a temporary and beneficial survival strategy, for example when bears eat many more calories than they require before hibernation. But it is fair to say that in humans, allostasis is both far more common and almost always harmful.

In 1993, two psychologists at Yale university, Bruce McEwen and Eliot Stellar, produced a paper which came up with a new term, known as allostatic load. They defined this as 'the cost of chronic exposure to fluctuating or heightened neural or neuroendocrine [related to the nerves and hormones] response resulting from repeated or chronic environmental challenge that an individual reacts to as being particularly stressful'.[12] In layperson's terms, if your background and genetics, and the life circumstances you face, make you particularly susceptible to stress, then that is likely to make you ill.

How? Let us count the ways. Hyperinsulinemia on its own, beyond the risks of it leading to diabetes, can harden the arteries, increase blood pressure, and is a factor in infertility – which we tackle in Chapter 8. Once it gets to allostatic load, things really take off. The longer-term risks of this include everything from an increased likelihood of certain cancers to the risk of bad dental health. Allostatic load has also been linked to a greater chance of heart disease, higher cholesterol and problems with bones and joints. Allostatic load is also linked to a shortening of the telomeres, the sort of end-caps to our chromosomes, which is an indication of biological ageing, as well as to greater frailty and a more rapid decline in cognitive function as the years progress.

All this is without mentioning one of the physical issues most closely linked to both chronic stress and insulin resistance: weight gain. This is so central that body mass index and waist-hip ratio – the latter a gauge of abdominal obesity – are among the potential markers for allostatic load. Weight, particularly in relation to stress, is a particularly complex area, and gets considered fully in Chapter 6.

Allostatic load is not something for which you can take a simple blood test, like type 2 diabetes. As much a descriptive theory as a phenomenon, it crosses the boundary between physiology and psychology, and can be identified by either discipline, for example biological markers or questionnaires filled in by patients.

Additionally, studies have shown an extremely strong correlation between allostatic load and things like low income or socioeconomic status, or where people live, education levels, ethnicity and other potential challenges, such as being a carer. This is not something which tends to strike without reason. More directly relevant to Hannah, who earns a good income, has a degree and has no caring or childcare responsibilities, other research has linked allostatic load to more difficult parental attachments in childhood. In something else that would strike a chord in Hannah, among the physical struggles and risks linked to allostatic load are poor sleep and potential chronic fatigue.

There are broader reasons why Hannah might be particularly affected. As a young woman, she faces societal pressure over her appearance, and particularly her weight, a common cause for stress in itself. But more than that, research has shown that attempts to lose weight using low-carbohydrate methods are also linked to increased cortisol. This is not the case for everyone, but as a phenomenon only recently uncovered by researchers it has potential repercussions for the multi-billion-dollar global industry based around the so-called keto diet and its many variants. It is something we will also explore in Chapter 6.

But one thing with Hannah's case history remains a puzzle, particularly to her. Given physical activity is so closely linked to insulin function and overall metabolic health, why is she not feeling the benefits from her regular and very high-intensity exercise regime? This is where our story takes an unexpected physiological turn.

The mystery of exertion

In a remarkably thorough piece of research, academics at the prestigious German Sport University in Cologne took thirty-two young men and very much put them through their paces. They were quizzed about their activity levels and physically tested, and thus classified according to fitness level. Everyone was fitted with a heart-rate-measuring watch plus a catheter to allow regular blood samples. Finally, in the time-honoured way for such studies, they were randomly split into two groups.

The first group underwent the Trier Social Stress Test, the sadistic-sounding laboratory method for artificially inducing stress via mock interviews and mental arithmetic tests that we heard about in the last chapter. The second group of volunteers were given what might sound like the less stressful option. This was a physical workout known as the Wingate test, also named after the place where it was devised, this time a sports institute in Israel. This involves sitting participants on a stationary bike and, after a warm-up, getting them to cycle at the maximum power and speed they can manage for thirty seconds, repeated four times and broken up with rest periods of slow pedalling. Finally, both groups were given a series of identical questionnaires, intended to gauge their own perceived stress levels.

The results were striking. A Wingate test is not easy – it is an all-out effort. Experienced researchers know to keep a bucket next to the stationary bike, as it can prove too much for some people. Nonetheless, the questionnaires very clearly showed the volunteers thought the mock interview was more stressful. But the cortisol levels told a very different story. These were not just higher in those who used the stationary bikes when they were actually cycling, but continued to rise, remaining notably more elevated than levels for the Trier test group well over an hour later.

The verdict was the same when stress was gauged another way, using the heart-rate monitors to measure a value known as heart-rate variability, or HRV – how much a person's beats-per-minute fluctuates over a time period. While the stereotypical idea of stress involves a racing heart, the opposite is true: a low HRV is seen as an indicator of greater stress. And once again, those who faced the physical task tended to record lower HRV values.

'It seems as if repeated physical stress activates the HPA axis more than the psychosocial stressor,' the researchers concluded – that is to say, the bike-based exertion set the body's stress response into motion more than the interview and tests. The stress effect for the intensive exercise, they added, seemed both stronger and longer-lasting than for the mental exercises.

Another finding was that the stress response in both groups did not seem to be lower for those who were fitter. Scientists have spent some time arguing about an idea called the cross-stressor adaptation hypothesis, which theorizes that repeated exposure to triggers of the HPA axis through exercise can help people cope with societal and personal stress. Some studies indicate it can – but this one did not.[13]

All this ties very neatly to Hannah. It is striking how closely the Wingate test imposed on the German volunteers resembles a compressed version of the sort of high-intensity exercise class Hannah attends several times a week, spending around £150 a month in fees to her upmarket gym in the process. High-intensity interval training, ubiquitously and more conveniently known as HIIT, is a hugely popular phenomenon in the exercise and gym world. It is popular because it is a very efficient form of exercise. Countless studies have shown that by pushing your heart near its maximum rate numerous, if brief, times, punctuated with rests, you become aerobically fitter while also decreasing your body fat and building muscle. The fact that the intensity increases your body's metabolic rate means the benefits can continue even after the exercise is over.

It is not clear whether HIIT achieves all these things better than more traditional, medium-intensity exercise, but it does do it in significantly less time, which has been enough to make what was once a niche phenomenon, used only by elite athletes, extremely popular. Originally known simply as interval training, it is by no means new, with Finnish coaches utilizing it for their Olympic contenders more than a century ago. It was, however, the extraordinary feats of another athlete which really made exercise scientists sit up and take note.

Often described as the greatest runner of all time, Emil Zátopek's primary claim to this accolade is his never-matched sweep of long-distance events in the 1952 Olympics, winning gold in the 5,000 metres, 10,000 metres and marathon. Famously garrulous and charming in all of the six languages he spoke, the Czech runner was beloved by fans for his never-say-die attitude on the track, one helped by a training regime which was both hugely gruelling and highly innovative. In later life, Zápotek recounted being mocked for his habit of sprinting 100 metres twenty times over, rather than the traditional preparation of longer, more plodding runs. 'Why should I practise running slow? I already know how to run slow. I want to learn to run fast,' he once said. 'Everyone said, "Emil, you are a fool!" But when I first won the European Championship, they said, "Emil, you are a genius!"'

Even the buoyant Zápotek ended up having much to be stressed about later in life. He championed democratic reforms in Czechoslovakia which were crushed in 1968, and was forced to spend years as a labourer away from his family. For obvious reasons we have no idea if his draining training regime hampered his ability to cope with the subsequent cortisol. But if it did, why might this be the case? It appears to be for the fairly straightforward evolutionary reason that pushing our body to its physical limit triggers a hormonal response mimicking what would have happened when our ancestors did the same thing, which for them would usually be to escape danger. When you hit 80 or 90 per cent of your maximum heart rate on a stationary bike, you are not in any peril beyond the mild risk of toppling off onto a foam mat in sheer exhaustion. But as we have seen, our HPA axis doesn't necessarily get the message. It still suspects we are running away from the hypothetical wolf.

The risk of so-called cortisol creep in high-intensity exercisers like Zápotek or Hannah is by no means uniform, but it does seem clear that intensity is the key. One study, which put volunteers through their paces at 40 per cent, 60 per cent and then 80 per cent of their aerobic capacity found that the increase in cortisol was notably greater for the latter two levels.[14] Other research has suggested that cortisol levels generally return to normal within twenty-four hours but that more rest might be needed, depending on both the person and the number of sessions squeezed in per week.[15]

Another apparent factor which is particularly relevant to Hannah's case is that the release of cortisol can depend in part on whether the exercise actually feels like fun. Studies have shown that if rats and mice are allowed to exert themselves voluntarily, for example using a wheel in a cage, their HPA axis is notably less triggered than when the exertion is forced on them, such as being made to swim in a tank. Humans are not laboratory rodents, but Hannah did say she sometimes felt compelled by guilt, or by worry about her weight and health, to take gym classes, and that in this mental state they felt almost like punishment.

There is, luckily, a relatively straightforward way to tackle the cycle of HIIT-induced cortisol creep: exercise less intensely and rest more. Research seems to show that even among elite endurance athletes, the shorter the break between training sessions, the more pronounced the rise in cortisol.[16]

What should Hannah do? Cut up her gym card, cancel the direct debit, forget about HIIT classes for ever? It is not as simple as that. High-intensity activity can bring benefits. One Spanish study carried out during the country's long Covid lockdown showed that people who did a daily bout of home-administered HIIT via squats and lifting weights showed, on average, fewer symptoms of depression than a group given a regime of medium-intensity exercise.[17]

Hannah's history with stress, as with all such examples in this book, is complicated, ongoing, and only ever partial. She began psychotherapy, to try and better understand the legacy of her earliest years. She also took up a couple of the more immediate practices we shall detail in Chapter 10, in particular working on improving her sleep and using a meditation app.

She was also advised to try a less strenuous exercise regime, but with one vital caveat – to remain active. That is perhaps the most confounding paradox of all. While, as we have seen, over-intense exertion can help push susceptible people further down the path of high cortisol, if someone is on the path towards prediabetes then one of the very best remedies they can undertake is to become active. High-intensity exertion on its own, separated from stress, has been shown to improve insulin resistance. Much depends on the person, and the circumstance.

Type 2 diabetes is largely an ailment of lifestyle, and in particular of lifestyles where people sit down a lot and barely exert their bodies. Research has shown that the tiniest physical movement, even standing up and walking around, particularly just after a meal, immediately helps your body to process blood sugars better. Virtually every doctor specializing in type 2 diabetes has a near-miraculous tale in which a long-term patient on several medications for the condition becomes markedly more active, whether through a job or other change of circumstance, and their diabetes goes into remission. Being active is key.

This apparent self-contradiction takes us back to the puzzle with which we began the chapter. Homeostasis in blood glucose is, in essence, a fairly simple process of balancing glucagon and insulin, and yet it so often can, and does, go wrong.

So why does it? This is where we must start to combine the two main threads of our story. Stress is in one sense nothing more than a product of hormones in various concentrations being fired around the bloodstream. But as we have also seen, particularly in the first two chapters, none of this happens in a vacuum. Both our propensity to produce greater or smaller amounts of cortisol and adrenaline at various times, and the way the body then responds to them, are the product of many factors, everything from the culture we live in to the upbringing that formed us within it.

It is in this latter direction that we shall now look, starting with those two vital and interlinked predictors of stress: status and work.

CHAPTER 5

Stress, Status and Work

As you might remember, the long-standing idea that stress at work was almost entirely a problem for the suited-and-tied male business executive was gradually and painstakingly debunked by a series of researchers. You might also recall that the final dismissal of this myth came in the early-1980s research of Robert Karasek, who concluded that the ideal recipe for a stressful job was in fact one where people had limited initiative or flexibility, but nonetheless high demands on their time and concentration. As we will see again and again in this chapter, stress is not generally created by high status. Quite the opposite: it is about a lack of control.

All this, it is fair to say, would come as no surprise to Anna. She started working in a vast consumer-goods warehouse four years ago, and knows full well what to expect from a shift there. Tasked with 'pre-sorting' orders which are then sent to a distribution centre, much of the work involves using the company's universal item sorter, a high-tech system which mixes robotics and artificial intelligence to shift vast numbers of packages to the right place.

'I grab a box from the line or a pallet, depending on which lines are open. I feed it into the robot and the robot actually sorts it,' she says. 'I have no control. I know I'm constantly under the watch of cameras. I have to feed the robots at a certain pace and if I stop they know, and how long for. If it's more than about five or ten minutes, I could be questioned about it.'

This monitoring allows Anna's bosses to total up her 'idle' time over the shift – which includes going to the toilet. 'In a ten-hour shift, if you go to the loo six times that can give you an hour of being "idle", when you're not,' she says. 'It's OK for me, but sometimes people have digestive problems or other health issues. In the summer, as well, people drink a lot of water to hydrate and that water has got to go somewhere.'

When Anna began at the warehouse as a temporary worker on nights, she found the pace – which she describes as 'A hundred miles an hour, just crazy' – very hard to take, not just mentally but also physically. 'It was very stressful and very exhausting. I'd get home in the morning and would struggle to stand up again once I got out of the car,' she says. 'My back was sore all the time from all the standing. You're not allowed to be caught leaning against anything, even if it gets quiet.'

Anna has not, as yet, taken a sequence of saliva swabs during the course of a shift to track her cortisol levels. But any expert on stress would be able to take a good guess at what the readings would be.

So why does Anna do it? Part of the answer is the pay, which is above what she would receive in many other similar roles. And now she is on staff and does day shifts, the set hours allow Anna and her partner to plan their working lives around their two primary-school-age children. Also, she receives holiday and sickness benefits. In her last job, working in logistics for a well-known British company, she would be sent home when work was quiet, being forced to use her holiday entitlement to cover this. If Anna had already taken an actual holiday she would subsequently have to work weekends or overtime to make up the hours. 'It can be stressful at the warehouse,' she says. 'But it's better than the last place.'

Just about every era seems to believe it faces an unprecedented burden of stress, from the mind-melting possibilities of rail travel and the telegraph in the Victorian age to the 1970s 'future shock' worries about the switch from an industrialized society to one based on information and disposability. Now people are having to deal with another revolution in work, much of it based around AI and other technologies, as well what seems to be a halt in previously rising living standards. To fill in the last forty or so years from Hans Selye's death, much of the modern discussion about stress has been connected to work, and virtually throughout that period there has been a recognition that you don't need to be in a senior job to suffer.

One major acknowledgement of the general impact of stress came with the UK's 1974 Health and Safety at Work Act, which said that as well as having a duty of care towards workers' physical well-being, employers needed to do the same for their mental health.[1]

One fascinating academic paper on the history of modern stress quotes a series of British people discussing the subject in the 1980s and 1990s for the Mass Observation project, an oral history of everyday life that ran from the 1930s to 1960s, before being revived in 1981.

'In the last month I have been prescribed mild tranquilizers as the doctor says I am suffering from "stress",' one female secondary-school teacher told the study in the mid-1980s, her deliberate emphasis indicating this was a slightly alien concept, even then.[2]

While the stereotype of stress being an issue exclusive to business executives had been dispelled, there remained a slightly macho residual approach to the subject. A *Sunday Times* article from 1985 purported to list sixty occupations in a 'stress league', from the most to least draining, with miners, police and construction workers at the top and nursery staff at the very bottom.[3] While no one would doubt that the first three can be difficult, the idea of nursery work being stress-free would only be credible to someone who has never met a toddler. It was most likely a product of this being a female-dominated profession.

So, how stressed are we now? The American Psychological Society publishes a particularly detailed annual survey of stress, based on large-scale polling. The most recent edition found that a quarter of all US adults said their stress level, on a scale of one to ten, was between eight and ten. The younger that people were, the worse the score seemed to be. Of those aged sixty-five plus, 9 per cent felt stressed at an eight-plus level; for adults under thirty-five, it was 34 per cent. Of this youngest cohort, 82 per cent said they had money worries. By many metrics, women and people from minority ethnic backgrounds appeared more stressed than average, as tends to be the case. And it was taking a toll. Two-thirds of people told the survey they had a chronic health condition, many which were associated with stress, for example high blood pressure or arthritis.[4]

The US is no outlier. An estimated 2.8 million Britons are on long-term sick-leave, many because of problems linked to stress. People in their twenties are considerably more likely than those in their forties to be out of work due to mental ill health.[5]

Is modern stress notably worse, or even especially different, from what people endured in the past? It depends in part on how you gauge things. On one level, life in twenty-first-century Britain has some very obvious advantages to that experienced by our Victorian ancestors, including a state-provided safety net, several decades' more life expectancy and a child mortality rate which is about sixty times lower. But stress is a many-layered phenomenon.

One of the researchers who has best understood and explained human stress is an American biologist called Robert Sapolsky, who in a slightly paradoxical twist has mainly achieved this by looking at animals. He spent over twenty years studying the complex social interactions of a troop of baboons in Kenya's Serengeti region, intermittently tranquillizing them with darts so he could take blood samples and measure their cortisol. Sapolsky is one of the best academic writers about any sort of science, and we will hear more about his research later in the book. But for now, consider his observation in an academic paper a couple of years ago which gave an overview of his four decades of studying stress. Among a list of what he called 'perhaps less obvious caveats and qualifiers' for the subject, he pointed to research showing that when it comes to how well various species cope with stress, much of it hinges on context.

'Stressors are less about the absolute intensity of a challenge than about its degree of discrepancy from the norm,' Sapolsky wrote. 'For a bird species migrating between the arctic and the tropics, dealing with intensely cold temperatures that, nevertheless, are precisely what would be expected, constitutes a normal workday in the arctic for the adrenocortical axis, whereas an unexpectedly chilly day in the tropics can be a life-threatening allostatic [stress-related] challenge.'[6]

This point is central when considering stress both as a modern phenomenon and an individual experience: it is not a competition. There will, inevitably, always be someone whose situation is objectively worse than your own, whatever the measure of stress chosen. What matters is the impact.

Stress and status

Presented with the details of Anna's working life, most people these days would probably agree it sounds stressful. But until quite recently, some experts would have simply advised her to get used to it.

In 1967, the British civil service's chief medical adviser, Daniel Thomson, was tasked with investigating the reasons behind fast-rising levels of sick-leave in the institution. After examining the illness records of a 5 per cent sample of 450,000 primarily desk-based officials of varying grades, Thomson and his team found that for all eight categories of sickness they looked at, lower-ranked staff took, on average, more time off than senior colleagues. Overall, the highest rank of civil servants, senior administrators, averaged 1.8 sick days a year; for the lowest, messengers, it was 12.7 days.[7]

This was a period when the UK was run by the resolutely modernizing Labour government of Harold Wilson, whose self-stated mission was to reshape the nation for the coming age. As such, you might have expected Thomson's conclusions to be followed by an effort to tackle this discrepancy in illness, perhaps to make the lower-grade jobs more amenable or stimulating. But while Thomson was a respected epidemiologist, he had other ideas. Civil servants, Thomson wrote, 'complain about the stress, strain and frustrations of modern living'. He went on: 'Many of these problems are, however, largely of their own making, because of their failure to reach emotional maturity and to become tolerant, patient and relaxed individuals, aware of their own limitations, having come to terms with their own surroundings, no matter how uncongenial.' Those stuck in low-grade, repetitive work should, he argued, 'accept [this] without a feeling of jealousy or grievance at other people's rather better luck', and acknowledge that some people are simply 'natural pace-makers and out-runners'. Officials in higher levels, he concluded, possessed 'different, and superior, physical characteristics', partly as a result of heredity.

If this did not already sound sufficiently Victorian, Thomson said that the greater average sickness rates among female civil servants was less a factor of their generally lowly roles – of 2,689 senior administrators studied, just 236 were women – than of 'divided loyalties' between work and family duties. Many female officials' sick leave days were taken to deal with domestic crises, Thomson declared, and as such they simply should be considered inefficient employees.

Coincidentally, a more modern approach to workplace stress also emerged from the English civil service, and in a study which had already begun by the time Thomson presented his report. It was led by Michael Marmot, the pioneering researcher into health-based inequalities who we encountered in Chapter 1. Starting in 1967, Marmot and his team tasked just over 17,500 male civil servants aged forty and older with filling in a questionnaire about things like smoking, medical treatments and leisure activities. For each man, the team also took an ECG reading of their heart and measured their blood pressure, cholesterol, body-fat percentage, height and weight. They then waited for a decade.

When this mass of information was correlated with records for subsequent deaths, the researchers found 'a steep inverse relation between grade and mortality' – that is, the more junior your job, the more likely you were to have died. Officials in the lowest seniority grade had three times the likelihood of death over the ten-year study period than those in the highest, and from any cause. Men in more junior grades were more likely to smoke but this only accounted for some of the difference.[8]

The report cited studies which linked chronic stress to illness but did not definitively connect the two. The fact that all causes of death were more common in junior roles 'might suggest the operation of one general factor in common to many diseases', Marmot and his team wrote, but said this could also be due to other factors, for example access to medical care.

Speaking now, just over forty years since the report known as *Whitehall One* was published, Marmot says that although he knew at the time about the 'high-demand, low-control' concept of job stress and had a good idea it might be involved in the findings, he felt that more research was needed.

This came with a follow-up study, also led by Marmot and inevitably known as *Whitehall Two*. It tracked more than 10,000 civil servants, many of them younger than the first cohort and now also including women. This confirmed the connection between lower-grade work and sickness, also noting how those in less responsible jobs tended to complain about job satisfaction and minimal latitude in how they went about their tasks. They were also more likely to rent rather than own their home and to have financial difficulties, both also strongly linked to stress.[9]

Whitehall Two and other studies irrefutably dispelled what Marmot now calls the 'ridiculous and self-serving idea that it's more stressful to be rich and high-status than to be poor and low-status.' He says: 'This whole idea of high-demand, low-control was a revelation. It's pretty awful to be low-status – you've got no control. And sure, if you're high-status, you tend to have more demand. But that's much more of your own choosing.'[10]

Given this knowledge, Marmot worries deeply about the sort of work carried out by people like Anna. 'It's as if we took everything we knew about psycho-social work hazards, put it in a syringe and injected people with it. And that's the nature of modern work for low-status people,' he says.

Even today, some still argue that stress caused by factors like jobs and income are, to a great degree, the responsibility of the person concerned. Unlike Daniel Thomson, they might not tell people to just get used to their station in life. Instead, they say, why don't they better it? This is no longer the Victorian age, the argument goes; everyone has access to education and healthcare – it's an equal contest. Such views are often heard, and felt, by people on the receiving end of stress. It can be a significant cause of guilt or shame. As ever, the reality is a lot more complicated.

Put simply, poverty and social deprivation, whether experienced as a child or as an adult, not only make stress and subsequent ill-health more likely but have the habit of trapping people in a cycle of self-reinforcement and shorter-term thinking which means it is much more difficult for them to escape. This happens in numerous ways, most not the product of conscious thinking, and in patterns set from the earliest days of infancy, or even the womb.

We will look in Chapter 9 at the complex subject of how very early childhood and pre-childhood events shape people's experiences of stress and how they respond to it. But when considering how hard it can be for adults to remove themselves from stressful situations, it is vital to take into account the words of Clyde Hertzman, a pioneering researcher into the impacts of adversity on child development: 'Early in life, the environment talks to genes and the genes listen.'[11]

A predilection to stress and thus chronic illness can hit people in three main ways, which often overlap. The first, sometimes called latent vulnerability, is Hertzman's idea about such dispositions being effectively embedded biologically during the crucial early months and years. Another way is cumulative – the adding-up of many years of adverse factors. A third, called the pathway model, notes how routes into stressful or unhealthy behaviours are often just followed, for example the much greater likelihood of a child with a parent who smokes or drinks to excess to do the same.

What does all this mean in practice? It means, to simplify only slightly, that life starts off as unfair and generally remains that way. For example, there is a mass of research showing that, on average, children from disadvantaged economic and social backgrounds tend to be less academically advanced before they start school. This is not a direct proxy for stress, but is very closely linked to it.

One famous US study found that the average vocabulary of three-year-olds from families with parents in professional jobs was roughly twice as large as that for their peers whose families received state benefits. Based on thousands of observed and recorded conversations, it compared children from a preschool in a US housing project with the offspring of academics in the same city who attended the university's in-house kindergarten.[12] The latter children, the report concluded, 'seemed to know more about everything'.

While this is both hugely important and widely demonstrated, correlations between poverty, life chances and stress, especially as measured by academic attainment, very clearly have the potential to create stigma. Michael Marmot recounts being told by one woman, 'That man Marmot is accusing me of being a bad mother, just because I'm poor.' His response – which Marmot admits is not entirely satisfactory – is that while the statistics are what they are, 'poverty is not destiny, and blame is unhelpful'.[13]

Stress is central to this process. Repeated studies have shown that, among schoolchildren, stress tends to be higher in those from families termed 'lower socioeconomic status'. This is also the case when the children simply perceive themselves to come from a lower socioeconomic background. Both the perception and the actuality make a difference.

This concept, sometimes referred to as identity salience, a slightly technical term for the centrality of how we see ourselves, is another reason why some people find particular situations more stressful than others: how our brains respond is based not just on who we are, but who we have been told we are. This can be a hugely powerful phenomenon.

One of the most fascinating and telling examples of this idea focused not on stress, or even poverty, but on another area rich with clichés and stereotypes: the idea that people from East Asian backgrounds tend to be good at maths, while women are less so. Researchers in the US recruited a cohort of Asian-ethnicity women undergraduates who were split randomly into three groups. All were asked to take the same maths test. Beforehand, each group were asked questions based on certain parts of their identity. The first were quizzed about their Asian heritage, for example whether their parents or grandparents spoke any languages other than English. The second group were asked about being women, such as whether they lived in a single sex or mixed part of the university campus. To serve as a control group, the last were asked about deliberately identity-neutral subjects, for example their views on various television networks.

The results were startling. Despite all three groups being of roughly equal academic ability, based on their university entrance scores, those asked to consider their Asian identity performed notably better in the maths test than did the control group, while the ones who had been thinking about their lives as women performed markedly worse.[14] This was identity salience in action. If you are repeatedly told a part of your identity shapes your life, it can happen.

Such stereotypes are particularly rife when it comes to poverty. When people were polled about how favourably or otherwise they felt towards an array of groups, including poor people and, listed separately, people who receive state benefits, they were consistently more negative towards the latter than the former.[15] Another project asked university undergraduates, a group generally viewed as quite socially open-minded, to rate the importance of twenty-two factors behind poverty. Those to which they gave the highest scores were all negative, notably that poor people are uneducated or lazy, or more likely to abuse alcohol or drugs.[16] This is a very powerful and hugely damaging set of societal assumptions to grow up with.

Given such attitudes, it is not at all surprising that living in economic insecurity tends to be a source of significant stress.

The Joseph Rowntree Foundation, a British charity that campaigns about poverty, recently produced a highly sobering report in which people were asked about a series of metrics related to stress, including lack of sleep, a sense of strain and the inability to focus. For all twelve metrics, people who rented their homes scored significantly higher than homeowners did. For ten of the measures, renters were on average twice as stressed. When the charity compared people who could pay all their bills with people who were struggling, the differences were even greater. Even more bluntly, the research found that the smaller someone's savings, the worse they slept.[17]

If this sounds rather simplistic, it is not. There is ample evidence that simply taking families out of poverty can have a hugely beneficial effect on stress, particularly for children's mental health. This was demonstrated, largely by accident, in one particularly illuminating study. This was intended to track the connection between long-term poverty and mental distress among children in the US state of North Carolina using the metric of diagnosed psychiatric symptoms. But mid-way through the research, something unexpected happened.

Some of the children being studied were from the Eastern Band of Cherokee Indians, a Native American community who live on a reservation in the state and which has legal autonomy from certain local laws, including on gambling. Mid-research, a casino opened on the reservation under a deal which granted every person living there a share of the profits plus first preference on jobs. This meant that about 15 per cent of children who began the study in families defined as poor were suddenly no longer poor.

When they were poor, these children had almost twice the incidence of diagnosed psychiatric issues as those whose families were better off. But after their incomes rose, levels of mental illness for the 'ex-poor' children fell to the same as the 'never poor'. In contrast, those who began poor and stayed poor did not see any improvement.[18] As Michael Marmot told the annoyed mother, poverty is not destiny. But it certainly tips the scales against you.

While some stereotypes about poverty are inaccurate – data

from England's NHS shows that higher-income people are the most likely group to drink potentially health-damaging amounts of alcohol[19] – research has nonetheless demonstrated that poorer and more stressed people tend to behave in ways that can reinforce poverty or ill health. This can include being less likely to complete a course of medicine and more likely to make financial decisions which, rationally, will not help them, such as playing lotteries and taking out very-high-interest short-term loans.

One very obvious explanation for this is sheer circumstance. If you are already comfortably off, then the idea of taking a one-in-roughly-50 million punt to win a lottery jackpot features less in your dreams. Similarly, poorer people often tend to be pushed towards more expensive payday-type loans because more mainstream forms of finance are not available to them.

But as we saw in Chapter 1, with the experiment about the impact on cognitive function of considering a hypothetical car repair bill, if someone is short of money in real life, the very state of being poor appears to create a 'scarcity mindset' in which looking beyond the most immediate problem becomes difficult. Researchers also sometimes call this the 'tunnel vision effect', where longer-term issues, including ones which could potentially relieve people's poverty or improve their stress and their health, are neglected.

This idea has been tested by psychologists through the innovative technique of getting people to play games, and making some of them 'poor' and others 'rich'. In one experiment, participants played a word-guessing game and were split randomly into two groups. The 'poor' cohort were allocated six guesses per round, while the 'rich' were given twenty. Those with fewer guesses, not unexpectedly, fared worse. But they also used notably more mental resources for the task, as shown by a post-game test of mental alertness – they were, as the researchers put it, 'depleted'. They had been forced to try harder for less reward.

Another test involved the groups playing a shooting-based video game, with the 'rich' given five times more shots per round than the poor. Once again, the shot-poor participants expended extra focus, taking notably longer than the rich to aim each shot. In another twist, some of the poor cohort were offered the chance to 'borrow' extra shots from a later round but at the price of losing two shots further on in the game, amounting to a 100 per cent rate of interest. This was, rationally, not a good deal. And yet some players took it up, and the researchers found that the longer someone took to aim each shot, the more likely they were to borrow.[20]

Excessive focus on immediate scarcity tended to result in neglect of the future. Poverty both creates stress and makes it harder to plot a route out of your predicament. It is a psychological, economic and then endocrinological vicious cycle.

The same research team who carried out the hypothetical car-repair experiment further demonstrated the cognition-sapping effect of deprivation with a real-world study of sugar cane farmers in southern India. The farmers receive the bulk of their annual income from the single cane harvest and can struggle to pay bills beforehand. Given a series of tests for cognitive function and reaction time, taken shortly before the harvest and then again after it had been completed, the farmers performed notably better on the second occasion, when money was more plentiful. As might be expected, when the farmers' stress levels were measured through heart rates and blood pressure, they were more stressed in the build-up to the harvest than afterwards. But even this stress didn't fully account for the differences in cognitive performance. There was an additional impact from what the researchers called 'attentional capture' – being too busy worrying about money to think about anything else.

'Being poor means coping not just with a shortfall of money, but also with a concurrent shortfall of cognitive resources,' the researchers concluded. 'The poor are less capable not because of inherent traits, but because the very context of poverty imposes load and impedes cognitive capacity. The findings, in other words, are not about poor people, but about any people who find themselves poor.'[21]

Dr Arif Rajpura, who is head of public health for Blackpool, a town in the north-west of England that has faced particularly ingrained problems of deprivation, stress and associated ill health, says he sees such effects reflected in his work every day. Rajpura dislikes the commonly-used term 'lifestyle factors' as reasons for stress and illness, as this implies an element of choice. 'Looking at these as individual behaviours is really simplistic,' he says. 'There are so many environmental factors that influence people's health and well-being – whether you've got enough money coming in, whether you've got a decent job, whether you've got friends, whether you live in a decent home. All of those basic tenets are so, so important.'

Blackpool, which has a population of around 140,000, has as many as 4,000 so-called homes of multiple occupation – houses or flats split into a series of individually rented rooms. These are cheap but involve people sharing a communal space with an often transient population of strangers, something studies have shown is often conducive to stress, and to poor mental health more widely.

Many of the solutions to Blackpool's issues are long term and involve central-government spending, for example improved schools and more early-years provision. But Rajpura does what he can, using an innovative approach to tackling more immediate health inequalities. One recent initiative has been to tackle the generally lower take-up of vaccines – such as the childhood combined jab for measles, mumps and rubella – among poorer families by sending vaccination teams directly to the homes of those least likely to come to a clinic appointment. Such non-attendees, Rajpura says, are not lazy or feckless; they just have too many other things to think about: 'There are so many complexities within our population. There are endless pressures with the cost of living, money, childcare, unemployment. So when a letter lands about vaccinations, it might not be a priority. There are bigger things going on in their lives.'

Being poor ages you

Persistent poverty and stress, as we have seen, can impede people's ability to plan well for the future. Unfortunately, there is even more bad news: being poor and being stressed can make you biologically older.

This has been shown by measuring people's telomeres, the tiny sequences of molecules that effectively act as a protective cap on chromosomes. These naturally become shorter as people age and their length is often used as a proxy for whether people's bodies are ageing more rapidly than a calendar alone would indicate.

One study in Glasgow, a city of particularly pronounced social disparities, found that if people's incomes were below £25,000 a year, their telomeres were particularly affected. Another marker for more rapid ageing was renting your home. The effect was, in telomere terms, roughly the same as from smoking or an unhealthy diet.[22]

Another study sought to examine the effect on telomere length of prolonged stress by measuring this in a group of healthy women, half of whom were carers to a family member and half who were not. Not unexpectedly, those who were carers said they were more stressed. However, simply being a carer did not necessarily mean shorter telomeres – it all depended on how long this had been going on. The more time a woman had been a carer, the shorter her telomeres.[23] Yet again, it is less about stress, as such, than stress as a long-term state.

Understanding stress and work

For many modern people, stress is a product of work. This basic fact has been understood for centuries, even if ways to combat it have proved more complex. Probably the first person to examine the field of what is now called occupational health was an Italian doctor called Bernardino Ramazzini, who spent years studying the ailments of various trades in seventeenth-century Modena, in the north of the country. Eventually compiled into a book, *De morbis artificum diatriba*, or *Diseases of Workers*, his studies chronicled both physical hazards like the continually hunched posture of a tailor or cobbler, and the mental exertion of the people he called 'learned men'. Ramazzini's work was very influential at the time, helping to limit the exposure to toxic substances in certain trades and winning very early compensation for some affected tradesmen.[24]

The formal study of workplace stress is a more recent innovation, with its origins in the early parts of the twentieth century, particularly following worries about sickness rates among factory workers during the First World War. For decades, as with Daniel Thomson's chastising words for junior civil servants, this was largely seen as the fault of individual workers. One 1950s study of absence among British coal miners and steelworkers, conducted by a pair of heavily Freud-influenced psychologists, saw them argue that persistent sick-leave was the result of employees projecting their own internal neuroses onto their bosses.[25]

Cary Cooper, the veteran professor of psychology, recalls the slow shift towards taking work-related stress seriously as a more holistic problem. 'When we became less of a manufacturing/engineering-based economy, and moved into a service-based economy, the problems people had were not with machinery . . . the problems people had were now with people,' he says.

Initially, Cooper adds, both unions and managers were sceptical about focusing on stress, but they are now largely on board – in part because the statistics are impossible to argue with.

'When you look at long-term sickness absence, historically it used to be muscular-skeletal diseases – back-ache and the like – that were the leading cause,' he says. 'And now, it depends which way you look at it, but anywhere between 52 per cent and 58 per cent of all long-term sickness absence is for stress, anxiety and depression. And when you go off with stress, you're off on average two to three times longer than if you get cancer.'

Reasons for stress at work vary, but they often come down to two main themes which intersect considerably: control and resources. Gail Kinman, professor of occupational health psychology at Birkbeck, University of London, has carried out numerous studies on the stresses faced by people in various professions, including social workers, prison officers, nurses and university academics.

'What work stress means to me is when you are in a situation where your resources don't allow you to fulfil the demands placed upon you,' she says. 'This isn't about a one-off challenge, but the accumulation of the hassles and the little problems that gradually wear you down.'

Even when people love their job, they can become hugely stressed if they are unable to do it properly. Much of Kinman's recent research has tracked British public sector workers during the post-2010 period known as austerity, when central and local government budgets were slashed, leading to an inevitable knock-on effect on public-sector staffing levels and budgets. To take one example, the prisons budget for England and Wales is now around £900m lower than it was in 2010, with about 10 per cent fewer staff and a correspondingly high turnover of employees – almost 15 per cent of frontline prison staff leave the service each year.

'Prison officers know what the job is,' Kinman says. 'They know that they're going to be dealing with dangerous people. But you expect to have the resources to help you. When I first started doing work about stress with prison officers, believe it or not I had grown, massive men coming up to me in the street in tears and saying, "Thank you so much for bringing to the public eye the work that we do, and the challenges that we have, because nobody really cares."'

Such stress, she adds, is particularly acute for people whose jobs involve them working directly with people, whether prison officers, teachers, social workers or nurses: 'Recovery is the massive thing. When you're unable to recover your resources, whether they're physical, psychological, or something like empathy, that's very hard.

For a lot of people I work with, compassion and empathy is kind of a commodity because they have to have it. But you can get what's called compassion fatigue.'

Much of this returns us to the findings of Robert Karasek all the way back in the 1980s – as we saw at the end of Chapter 2 – that workplace stress tends to be a product of the demands placed on people and the amount of personal autonomy they can exercise. If you are a prison officer, social worker or nurse who spends each shift racing from crisis to crisis amid a lack of staffing, then as well as the sheer increase in demands on your time, any professional leeway is necessarily restricted by sheer circumstance.

The wider psychology behind stress and a sense of control is utterly fascinating. One famous 1971 study exposed people to increasingly unpleasant volumes of jet-engine noise, with the test subjects instructed to let staff know when it became too much. One group was given access to a switch which they were informed would limit the volume. Despite the fact that the switch was connected to precisely nothing, the impression of control meant this group tolerated, on average, roughly twice the noise levels of those not given a switch.[26]

If this all sounds very primal, it is. Another well-known test saw the same thing done to rhesus monkeys, with their cortisol levels monitored. The monkeys who believed they could control the noise with a lever experienced notably lower stress levels.[27]

Is my job stressful?

Peter writes: Deciding how stressful a job is depends on many factors, and it is, very clearly, often a personal thing. So, let's look at our own examples. In my case, as a politics journalist in the UK, a role I started in 2016, the years post-Brexit have certainly ticked the box labelled 'High demand'. There is almost always a lot going on, and it has to be covered. Sometimes it involves working late – crucial parliamentary votes can run well into the evening – and requires weekend work and travel. Time with friends and family can suffer.

But on the other side of the equation, there is control. Ultimately, news editors decide which stories we reporters cover, but it is a collaborative process. And apart from periods of particularly frantic news, there are always parts of my working day where it is entirely up to me what I do. Sometimes I meet an MP or an official for coffee or lunch to get information for future stories. At other times I make plans for new projects, or even spend ten minutes staring into space to think. I'm trusted to make good use of my time. Finally, I work with a small and highly collaborative team, where we all help each other. Sometimes it's very busy and yes, it can be stressful. But the stress is usually stimulating. I'm very lucky, and I realize it.

Richard writes: I'm in a lucky position. I essentially govern what I do on a daily basis. I manage a busy laboratory group and we tackle current research questions that are important to most of us in society. I enjoy improving our understanding of how human metabolism works in both health and disease. We know very little about this field and it's an exciting time to be working in this area.

Yet even a perceived perfect job has drawbacks. Trying to obtain research funding in a non-Oxbridge university is very challenging and can be stressful. It can take two or three years to formulate a good research idea, prepare the ethics application and write it, only for the funding application to fail. There is also the pressure to publish our research findings in the best possible journals within our respective research area. This process can also take years to achieve and is littered with editor- and peer-review hurdles. All this said, it is still an enjoyable field to work in and I am able to translate the findings in the laboratory to help people understand their individual metabolism and improve their health.

Even when it comes to ideas of demand and control, workplace stress is never a static process. It is now nearly eighty years since the head of manufacturing at Ford introduced the word 'automation' to the English language, and today, with rapid developments in technology, particularly artificial intelligence, a whole new series of worries have arrived. These include the much-discussed idea that AI could simply do away with the need for humans in many roles. Even now, communication technologies have revolutionized many desk-based jobs, with the Covid pandemic accelerating the recognition that a lot of these could, with a few tweaks, be done from home.

Homeworking can very obviously, at times, be a way to relieve stress. This is especially true for people with caring responsibilities, who can, for example, do a school pick-up and then finish off work emails in the kitchen, as the family dinner cooks in the oven. For people with long and tricky commutes – increasingly common when many younger people are priced out of big cities – being able to work from home a couple of days a week can be a blessing. But it is not straightforward.

Another impact of Covid was that some companies realized they could save money by either dispensing entirely with physical offices or scaling back the amount of space. Younger and more junior employees, in particular, can suffer from near-constant homeworking, if it is not what they want. Apart from missing out on learning from others, working with a laptop on your bed, because you live in a cramped, shared home, is far from ideal.

Gail Kinman says that homeworking can be particularly hard in professions with a heavy emotional load, for example social workers, who spend part of their day visiting clients, sometimes in very distressing situations. A big element of their support system is the opportunity to collaborate, commiserate and otherwise just talk with colleagues in an office. During Covid, when this was not possible, Kinman says, some social-worker teams would start a mass Zoom call in the morning and just keep it running. Even if no one was talking, the sense of companionship, even the click of someone else's computer keyboard, felt reassuring and relaxing.

A few companies have combined a push to homeworking with sometimes alarming efforts to monitor staff remotely, often using highly intrusive technology. In his job as a journalist, Peter was contacted a couple of years ago by an employee of Teleperformance, a global corporation which provides call centre staff to other companies. Teleperformance had just told its UK workers it would introduce a new monitoring system for home-based staff where they would have to click a 'break mode' in an app to explain why they would not be at their desk even momentarily, for example to fetch water or go to the toilet.[28]

More alarmingly, the company also said staff would be monitored by webcams to check whether they were eating or looking at their phones when they were meant to be working. Infractions would be judged by AI, with images sent to a manager for possible disciplinary action. After objections from trade unions and politicians, the webcam plan was dropped for the UK, but is now being used for staff in other countries.

Such technology has become increasingly prevalent, according to Andrew Pakes, who was deputy general secretary of the trade union Prospect and is now a Labour MP. He has a particular interest in the changes to modern workplaces and the stresses these bring. His research has uncovered more than 500 apps and products on sale to digitally monitor staff, some with names like *Sneak* and *Spy Agent*. Many are not legal in the UK, he says, yet it is a growing area. 'One of the big challenges in technology – and it's been boosted by flexible work – is that because managers feel like they can't walk up and down an office and physically check on people, they want tools to make sure they are present and contributing,' he says.

More widely, Pakes argues, there is a need to make sure that existing technologies like email do not cause the boundaries between work and home to be overly blurred, making it harder for staff to switch off from workplace stress. 'If you were cooking tea for your kids at 6 p.m. on a Friday and your employer banged on the door, sat down at the table and pushed the plates away, saying, "How's this project doing?", clearly we know that's abusive,' he says. 'But we're allowing the psychological, digital version of that with emails coming into people's inboxes. That can still cause pressure. Younger employees might feel the need to respond quickly, in case they don't get promoted. And you might have someone with caring responsibilities who might feel they're missing out on an opportunity because they can't do what others are doing.'

The rise of AI has been presented by some as a possible boon for work stress: let the computers take care of the tedious, high-demand/low-control work, while the humans focus on the creative stuff, or, in some versions of this future vision, relax into a three-day working week. However, this might not necessarily be the case.

Dr Abigail Gilbert is co-director of a think-tank called the Institute for the Future of Work, which, as the name suggests, researches how employment is likely to change amid the technological revolution and how this can be done more effectively and fairly. She points to the difficulties posed by something called Moravec's Paradox, devised in the 1980s by a group including the eponymous Hans Moravec, an Austrian computer scientist. This states that when it comes to robotics and AI, it is relatively easy for a machine to undertake complex reasoning tasks, but it will often struggle with certain things which are very basic for a human, notably visual perception and motor skills. 'If I was going to look after my grandmother, and I had to bend down to pick up a plate, and then help pick her up, that would be really complicated for a machine. However, it's quite easy for AI to sift CVs,' Gilbert explains.

One real-life example of this phenomenon is the way that self-driving cars and lorries have still not yet truly arrived. Instead, one part of driving which computers have taken over is navigation, meaning the highly skilled 'Knowledge' of London black-cab drivers, painstakingly learned over years, is arguably defunct. 'We're at the point where the mechanical side of driving is more important to be done by a human than the cognitive side of the work,' Gilbert says. 'Here, technological augmentation is a kind of de-skilling.'

And so, as with Anna in her warehouse, or Teleperformance staff being monitored by webcam, for some people this new era of work could become doubly stressful: largely repetitive, and at the same time with any personal autonomy crushed by the monitoring of AI algorithms. 'We don't have to think that it is inevitable,' Gilbert says. 'There are different types of policy intervention that could prevent this. A really important one is requiring employers to undertake good work-impact assessments before they adopt technologies, to think about how to steer innovation towards approaches that also advance the social good, as well as allowing them to secure productivity gains.'

Some countries are thinking about this more carefully than others. While the UK's health and safety laws remain mainly focused on physical harm in a traditional workplace, Gilbert says, the EU is drafting regulations on what are known as 'psycho-social harms', such as stress.

These are complex and evolving issues, taking in corporations, unions and governments from around the world. But that will be of limited comfort to anyone feeling the impact of a lack of control over their job, or unceasing, intrusive demands on their time and energy.

One of the curiosities of stress, particularly that connected to work, is that sometimes the first tangible sign of its cumulative effect comes in the waistline, or on the scales. Is this simply a function of not having enough time to cook or shop properly? That can often be a factor. But when it comes to stress and weight, there is a lot more to it – as the next chapter shows.

CHAPTER 6

Carbohydrates, Appetites and Stigma: Stress and Weight

If stress as a whole can never be fully understood outside the wider context in which it exists, the same is true tenfold when it comes to obesity and body shape. There is an important and fast-emerging scientific narrative to be told about how stress can affect our weight, but it can only be properly explained if you acknowledge that this is a subject containing endless social and cultural pitfalls. Perhaps the most important of these is stigma, and when it comes to body shape, this can affect pretty much anyone. Consider the case of Andrej.

Andrej is twenty-six and plays as a midfielder in the top division of a European football league. His is not a name you would necessarily know unless you were a fan of the particular team, while the league in which he features is not among the continent's absolute elite. But by more or less any metric, he enjoys the sort of professional sporting career that millions of young people dream about and only a handful achieve.

He was a settled and valued member of the first team, playing most weeks. His income, around average for the league as a whole, put him in the top 0.2 per cent of taxpayers for that country. Money would never again be a problem. Andrej was also happy – he was doing well, scoring regularly, loved by the fans.

But then the goals started to dry up. Andrej, normally a bustling and physical presence on the pitch, seemed flat, diminished. He was substituted, then dropped for a period. The club's doctors were puzzled. He was not injured; he just seemed to have lost his zest. The answer came amid a general physical check, when Andrej was weighed. He had lost 4kg. Tests of his muscular strength showed readings markedly lower than in pre-season. Was he ill? The answer, eventually given by a sheepish Andrej to the team doctors, was more straightforward, yet also more surprising: he had been on a diet.

Andrej has the type of footballers' physique familiar to those who might remember the English striker Wayne Rooney's playing days: not hugely tall but broad, barrel-chested and extremely strong. One of Andrej's great abilities on the pitch had been the way he could almost brush defenders away, his low centre of gravity and powerful core making it hugely difficult for them to tackle him. Andrej knew all this. But he felt his body looked chunky next to the more obviously lithe, toned torsos in the dressing room. If you put Andrej in a pair of trunks on a packed beach, he would be very obviously lean, muscular and athletic compared to almost anyone else. But this was not the comparison he was using. And so, he told the team doctors, he went on a diet. Suddenly he was no longer the same player.

Take another example. Ellie came to Richard's clinic because she was worried about an irregular menstrual cycle and aching joints. Her blood glucose and cortisol were both in the higher range of what is normal and there were signs she might be on the road towards insulin resistance, where the hormone stops working efficiently. Ellie accepted that she was stressed. She described the time demands of her job in finance as 'sometimes mental', particularly when added to worries about a sibling with intermittent depression. But one thing was particularly striking about Ellie's first visit to the clinic. Among the standard measurements recorded are height and weight. Ellie refused the latter. 'I don't really want to know what it is,' she said. 'It changes all the time anyway.' It later emerged that she was also seeing a psychotherapist to try to understand previous issues with binge eating. Ellie was a self-confessedly voracious consumer of social media and, like Andrej, was consistently comparing herself to others who she just thought looked better.

If you were to take an entirely random group of people from the street and quiz them on how they felt about their weight and their bodies, variants of these sorts of stories would be depressingly common. Depending on how the question is framed, something around 20 per cent of all British people confess to disliking their bodily appearance, even feeling ashamed of it. For teenagers this proportion is nearly a third.

Even when viewed as an entirely biological phenomenon, weight can be hugely complicated. But one thing is clear: nothing is ever improved by making people feel guilty, or ashamed or stigmatized. This chapter is not a guide to losing weight. If there are a lot of titles out there about stress, that is nothing compared to the miles of shelves stacked with diet books. Many of these contain perfectly sensible information. But at the same time, studies indicate that fewer than one in ten dieters who lose weight keep it off in the longer term. This is not some mass failure of human will. When it comes to weight, the biological, social and political odds are stacked against us.

The idea of what is called an obesogenic environment, one in which gaining weight becomes almost the default, is not new. But the sheer amount of evidence for its effects is striking.

A series of studies have confirmed the close relationship between the number of takeaway food outlets in an area and the chance a local person will be overweight, one exacerbated by the way that unhealthy snacks can now be summoned with the click of an app. A very recent piece of research tracked the correlation between children's weight, body-fat levels and signs of inflammation, and factors including the proportion of so-called ultra-processed foods – broadly defined as the sort of thing you couldn't conjure up in a domestic kitchen – sold in local shops and a lack of nearby public green space.[1]

The factors behind obesogenic environments have been building for many decades and involve things as fundamental as urban design and transport options. Another element is the implacable power of major food manufacturers, whose influence can be seen in any supermarket, their aisles stacked with highly caloric but nutritionally empty products. What government pushback exists has tended to begin modestly before getting watered down even more after corporate lobbyists argue about consumer choice. The UK government has spent years planning to ban so-called multi-buy deals on foods doused with fat, salt or sugar, but at the time of writing, it has not happened.

Just over a quarter of English adults are now obese, while two thirds are above what is seen as a healthy weight. Obesity statistics for children as they leave primary school are roughly similar.[2] These statistics are broadly reflected in many other wealthier countries, and in pretty much all of them the trend is sharply upward. Crucially, you are more than twice as likely to be obese if you live in a poorer area than in a richer one. It cannot be said enough times: this is not a fair fight.

What can this chapter offer you? Thanks to a mass of emerging research it can bring an extra perspective, and an important one. Stress is, in its own way, a significant part of the issue of weight. We have already seen that an HPA axis on continually high alert and the cortisol levels that come with this can cause a feedback loop of elevated insulin and blood sugars, with consequences for how fat is processed and stored. But stress also plays a huge role in the other side of the equation. Research shows very strongly that people who are stressed are likely to eat more overall, and to be drawn towards unhealthier foods. In turn, if someone is unhappy with their weight or body shape, that can be a source of significant stress. It is all connected.

Let us start with the very basics. What makes a body increase in weight? As with much connected to this subject, it depends in part on what question you ask.

The caloric conundrum

The idea of obesity as we now understand it was first set out by Jean Mayer, a French-born physiologist who started to examine the societal reasons behind slowly increasing weight levels in the US in the 1950s, when being overweight was still generally dismissed as some sort of moral failure. Along with advising UN organizations on how to help people who simply did not have enough food, Mayer carried out pioneering research into why others, in richer countries, were seemingly eating too much.

Born in Paris in 1920, Mayer's life had already been extraordinary before he reached America. He was captured by the Germans in 1940 while fighting to protect British troops being evacuated at Dunkirk, but escaped from a prisoner-of-war camp and joined the French Resistance. He then became a British agent, seeing further action in North Africa and Europe before working on General Charles de Gaulle's staff in London. He ended up with more than a dozen decorations, including the Croix de Guerre and the Legion of Honour.

After the war, Mayer moved to the US, studied at Yale and became so respected a nutritionist that he advised three successive presidents – Richard Nixon, Gerald Ford and Jimmy Carter. Among his discoveries was the fact that while people tend to eat more food after physical exertion to compensate for the calories they have burned, the opposite is generally not true – if someone becomes gradually less active, their appetite rarely diminishes to match. This creates what Mayer termed a 'continued positive energy balance', and thus weight gain, a wider idea that became known as the energy balance model.

This positive balance does not have to be significant. One calculation has suggested that if someone is regularly consuming just ten calories a day above what is termed their weight-maintenance energy requirement, they will gain about half a kilo a year. This is, in fact, a common trajectory for many middle-aged people. Mayer's argument was that since teaching yourself to eat less is notoriously difficult, you should instead become more physically active, levelling up the energy balance from the other side. This is, however, not easy in an obesogenic environment.

While reiterating that this is not a diet book, one important if slightly self-contradictory point needs to be noted. For all that Mayer was, and remains, correct that lower levels of physical activity appear to have played a significant role in the global spread of obesity, this does not automatically mean that simply going to the gym or for a run will make you slimmer. Even setting aside the risk that high-intensity exercise could increase your cortisol levels, as experienced by Hannah in Chapter 4, the physiological calculations are simply not on your side. Or to put it in the slightly more blunt way used – generally in private – by public health experts: 'You can't outrun a Mars bar.'

This comes down to simple caloric maths. It's relatively straightforward to become active enough to make up for a ten-calorie daily surplus and thus maintain your weight. But trying to exercise your way to a consistently lower weight is tough. To use the above comparison, there are about 240 calories in a current standard-size Mars bar. The calories burned up in exercise vary significantly, depending on factors including the intensity of the activity and the person involved, but a fairly broad rule of thumb is that jogging accounts for about 100 calories per mile, so to make up for one standard-size bar of chocolate, someone would need to go for a half-hour run at a decent pace. Alternatively, walking briskly for an hour would do it. And that's just for one, smallish-sized snack. Before too long, there are not enough free hours in the day.

A fascinating illustration of this conundrum came in a study carried out by researchers in the early 1980s in then-communist Bulgaria; one which for all sorts of reasons could probably never be replicated today. It involved a group of overweight women who, over the forty-five-day course of the experiment, lost an average of 12.4kg each. That happened despite them eating nearly 2,800 calories a day, well above the 2,000-calorie daily intake currently recommended for women.

How did they manage it? Well, this is where the twist comes. The women were put through an exercise regime which, if imposed on people who had not volunteered, might breach several minor clauses of the Geneva Convention. Their daily programme lasted ten hours and included gymnastics, swimming, tennis, athletics, dancing and long-distance running races, capped with a weekly walk that was initially 20 kilometres – slightly over 12 miles – then increased by 5 kilometres each week. The women each expended an average of 3,700 calories per day – more than many professional sportspeople. It was definitely effective, but not exactly easy to incorporate into everyday life.[3]

None of this is to suggest that being more active is a bad idea. In pretty much any circumstances, a greater amount of physical activity will make you healthier, whether or not it changes the numbers on a set of scales. It is also very likely to improve your mental health and cognitive function, and might make it less likely you get dementia when older, something scientists believe is connected to the work of myokines, the mysterious proteins produced by the skeletal muscle system.

With all those caveats and qualifications noted, let's get on with explaining the complex interactions of stress and weight.

The various theories of weight

In the most basic physiological terms, too much stress, and the hormonal consequences of that state, can play havoc with the way your body processes, uses and stores fat. As we saw in Chapter 4, the reason for this is primarily to do with insulin.

To reiterate the basic process: cortisol releases stored glucose, intended to be burned up as we respond to what our HPA axis believes is an immediate and possibly existential threat. If this glucose is not, after all, consumed in something like a half-mile sprint back to the safety of a cave, it creates elevated blood sugar, which in turn requires an uptick in insulin levels to rebalance things. The body now has a higher level of insulin and potentially increased cortisol, a state which if repeated chronically can lead to insulin resistance, in which the hormone works less efficiently.

What is also important for this chapter is the way that elevated insulin affects fat processing. Fat cells are not just inert storage. As well as being a reservoir for energy they are an active endocrine organ, influenced by all sorts of hormones and other bodily secretions. And one of the effects of too much insulin is that it inhibits lipolysis. Lipolysis is the process whereby fat stored in the body as triglycerides, the most common type of bodily fat, is broken down to the less complex glycerol and free fatty acids, both of which can be used for more immediate energy use. The fact that insulin affects lipolysis has been known for decades, but we now also understand how this happens. To get briefly technical, when insulin binds to receptors in fat cells it reduces the levels of a cellular messenger which forms part of the phosphatidylinositol kinase-3/protein kinase B pathway, usually shortened to the PI3K/AKT. Imbalances of the PI3K/AKT pathway are associated with all sorts of difficulties, including possible type 2 diabetes, as well as other inflammation-connected ailments, and heart disease. In this particular case, less lipolysis results in slower fat breakdown and more fat storage – something which becomes notably worse if fat cells become resistant to insulin, which, as part of the endocrine system, they can.

However, this is just one instance – one of the many complications of endocrinology is that the same hormone can have different effects on different parts of the body, and also if other hormones are in the mix. Studies have shown that cortisol can actually increase lipolysis – but seemingly only in the presence of insulin, and only in subcutaneous fat. The same phenomenon of cortisol-boosted lipolysis has been demonstrated in mice via a somewhat grim-sounding laboratory experiment in which mice showing submissive behaviour were put in cages next to ones who appeared dominant. For twenty minutes every day, partitions between the cages were raised, forcing the meeker animals to interact with the more bullish ones, as a deliberate means of increasing stress hormone levels in the submissive group. The researchers saw a 'profound' impact on the lipid metabolism of the stressed mice, including notably higher levels of cholesterol in their blood.[4]

This is by no means the end of the process. Other studies have linked consistently high glucocorticoids, the group of hormones including cortisol, with a particular propensity to storing fat around the stomach, something which has health impacts of its own, including yet more risk of type 2 diabetes and an elevated chance of heart disease. This effect on fat distribution is very obviously demonstrated by the way that abdominal obesity is one of the signs of Cushing's syndrome, when the body manufactures too much cortisol for reasons other than stress.

A particularly worrying weight-related effect of chronic stress was also observed in the unfortunate mice: it had a notable effect on their livers. A surfeit of glucocorticoids in our system can cause something called de novo lipogenesis, a sort of reverse lipolysis in which the body builds new fat from sugar and proteins. This has a tendency to build fat around the liver in particular. Non-alcoholic fatty liver disease, as this becomes if left unchecked, can be very serious, with effects including high blood pressure and type 2 diabetes. In the very worst cases it can lead to cirrhosis, the long-term liver damage which can be fatal. All this is alarming enough, but it is only half the story. This is very much a circular process – a malfunctioning metabolism creates a tendency to put on weight, but then in turn, greater weight has a tendency of its own to push us ever further from homeostasis.

One of the biggest factors here is the notion that different types of fat do not act in the same way. So-called adipose fat, the deposits around someone's stomach and organs, is notably more reactive to cortisol than standard subcutaneous fat – that which is stored under the skin. The impact of cortisol in the body is controlled by an enzyme that makes the hormone active, and there are higher levels of this enzyme in abdominal fat.

The more you look at the connections between stress and weight, the harder it becomes to disentangle cause and effect. We know that high cortisol appears to cause people to put on weight around their waist. However, other experiments have shown that people with a tendency to this so-called apple shape appear to be more prone to stress in the first place. One US study showed that when a group of women were put through an artificial stress situation, those with a larger waist-to-height ratio perceived the situation as being more threatening, and performed worse in cognitive tests, compared with women with proportionately slimmer waists. This effect was observed even if the more apple-shaped women were slim. It was the distribution that mattered, not the amount.[5]

One of the clearest examples of this intermingling of causes and symptoms is the way that chronically elevated cortisol, in the presence of insulin, not only makes fat deposits more likely, almost regardless of how much food you have eaten, but can also change the way people eat in the first place. Numerous laboratory experiments have echoed what many people experience in real life: being stressed is likely to make you eat more and eat less healthily. In part this can be just circumstantial. If you are awash with work tasks and get home late, a takeaway pizza will be significantly more appealing at 9 p.m. than cooking a meal from scratch. The same thing will most likely be true if the stress comes from something which simply occupies all your mental foreground, leaving no space for planning meals. But physiology plays its part.

There is an entire sub-genre of academic studies in which volunteers are placed under artificial stress and then presented with a table of various foods and told to snack as they please. Thinking the experiment is over, they graze away, not realizing that every morsel is being noted. Each time, those exposed to stress gravitate towards fatty, sweet or salty choices, and eat more overall than the control group, who were not stressed. One British university recruited volunteers for a version of this research by placing adverts around the campus saying the only qualifications were 'liking chocolate and having the ability to eat it with no adverse side effects'. Unsurprisingly, they recruited enough test subjects.[6]

The reasons for this are complex and not entirely understood. One important part of the process seems to be the fact that glucocorticoids such as cortisol have an effect on the hypothalamus, and on another part of the brain called the mesolimbic pathway, both of which are closely linked to reward and craving. They also seem to inhibit the function of leptin, a hormone released by fat tissues which plays a central role in telling your brain when you are full. Under stress, cortisol can also seemingly trigger the release of two other substances, corticotropin-releasing hormone (the main regulator of the stress-hormone HPA axis) and neuropeptide Y (which plays a key role in homeostasis), both of which have been shown to stimulate appetite.

Yet another idea is the fascinating concept known as 'selfish brain theory'. The brain is unlike other organs, not least in that it consumes about 20 per cent of bodily energy just to tick over, despite being about 2 per cent of our body weight. It is also the orchestrator of all homeostatic processes and is entirely reliant on blood sugars, being barely able to store any of its own energy. The theory surmises that the brain will always prioritize its energy needs above anything else, and that in times of stress it may seek to make sure bodily reserves are well stocked up, even if this has a negative long-term impact on the waistline.

Whatever the cause, as with everything else connected to stress, it does not affect everyone in the same way. A variety of experiments have shown that stress, whether imposed in a laboratory or recorded from the outside world, tends to make about two thirds of people hyperphagic, the technical term for them eating more. The other third eat as normal under stress, or in some cases lose their appetite. Stress-connected weight loss is notably less studied than weight gain, for two reasons. The first is that it tends to be much less common. The other is because, beyond rare and extreme cases, losing weight is easier to address and brings fewer potential long-term health consequences.

> ## Why some and not others?
>
> Why do some people react to stress by eating less well, but others don't? There is no single answer but part of it seems to be, as ever with stress, rooted in childhood, particularly in early childhood.
>
> A study of more than 3,000 Dutch six-year-olds found that those with the highest readings of cortisol in hair samples were nearly ten times as likely to be obese than those who did not.[7] This same association between high cortisol and being overweight or obese has also been demonstrated in adults. Other research has shown that children who are obese seem to have particularly elevated cortisol levels late in the evening, when under the normal diurnal slope it should be well on the way towards its lowest point as sleep begins, a particularly worrying dysfunction.
>
> As we have seen, a childhood marked by high cortisol does not automatically mean difficulties at home or elsewhere in life, but there is very often a correlation. Much as with stress as a whole, the potential impact on weight seems connected to wider life circumstances. One striking British study tracked more than 6,000 people for a decade and found that the people who said they had the fewest close relationships, or others in whom they could confide, were the most likely to gain weight over that period.[8]

One theory as to why stress-eaters tend to reach for starchy or sweet foods goes back to the idea of pure ease: if you're in a rush, or distracted, then quick, convenient ways to fill yourself up tend to be less healthy. But there does seem to be more to it. Recent worries over ultra-processed foods, which are almost always high in refined carbohydrates, fats, sugars, or a combination of some or all of these, has prompted a mass of new research into their seemingly addictive properties. Such foods, generally defined as factory-created items which you could not reproduce in an average home kitchen, are usually very dense in calories. But there is another feature which appears to make them addictive for some people.

In nature, foodstuffs tend to be high in fat, or in carbohydrates, but rarely both. For example, an apple has a proportion of carbohydrates to fat of 36:1. A piece of salmon might have three-quarters of its calories in fat, but virtually no carbohydrates. In contrast, ultra-processed foods tend to be packed with both – and this appears irresistible. A chocolate bar, for example, often has a near 50:50 mix. Some fast foods even manage an equally irresistible near three-way split between fat, carbohydrates and protein, for example breadcrumb-coated fried chicken. Some of these highly appealing ultra-processed foods can even pose as being healthy, for example 'protein bars', which also contain notably more fat and sugar than you might expect, not to mention nearly twice as many calories than the hypothetical Mars bar from earlier.

A recent British study found people seem to be especially drawn to foods with a roughly equal carbohydrate–fat ratio, and that simply being processed did not in itself make them more appealing.[9] Another draw seems to be that the fats and starches in artificial foods are generally easier for your body to break down, bringing swifter gratification.

Finally, it has been shown that ultra-processed foods can prompt a response in your brain from dopamine, the neurotransmitter central to a sense of reward, similar to that created by tobacco, alcohol, or drugs. It is no surprise they can seem addictive.

The paradox of global weight gain

All this gives plenty of hints about why some people gain weight when stressed, while at the same time offering depressingly few solutions. However – to reiterate what is becoming the trademark refrain of this chapter – it is only part of the picture.

One perhaps surprising element is that while most people might assume we eat considerably greater quantities than people did a generation or two ago, the evidence for this is distinctly mixed. It appears to be possibly the case for Americans. Research based on US census data worked out that the average American adult now consumes nearly 2,500 calories a day, 20 per cent more than their peers in 1970, with a diet containing less sugar but notably more high-fructose corn syrup, a ubiquitous commercial food sweetener.[10] In contrast, a study of food consumption in England between 1980 and 2013 calculated that total caloric intake had actually fallen.[11]

How could this tally with the very obvious increase in obesity? One slightly unnerving hypothesis is that Jean Mayer's ninety-year-old energy balance model has simply gone out of date. This sounds almost impossible to believe: the one thing most people would claim to understand about weight is that if you eat less and move more, you will stay slim. The response is: well, yes and no.

In yet another blow for already put-upon younger generations, there is evidence that gaining weight is just easier to do nowadays. This was shown when scientists analysed several decades of survey responses from Americans about their food intake and physical activity levels. It found that while overall caloric intake had gone up by 10 per cent or so, leisure time activity levels had also risen. When everything was crunched together and various other demographic factors were taken into account, they concluded that if a modern person followed exactly the same dietary and exercise regime as someone from the mid-1990s, they would somehow end up about 10 per cent fatter. The researchers suggested a series of possible reasons, including chemicals in food, the impact of the widespread use of antidepressant drugs, even changes over time to people's stomach microbes caused by things like antibiotics in meat.[12]

A more holistic counter-theory to Mayer's idea is known as the carbohydrate-insulin model of obesity. This proposes that when it comes to the modern era, the energy balance model might be looking at things the wrong way round. Rather than Mayer's notion of people being in energy surplus and thus storing fat, the carbohydrate-insulin model takes as its starting point the metabolic response to a diet heavy in carbohydrates, particularly ones which break down quickly in the body, known as having a 'high glycaemic index'. Eating a lot of rapid-action carbohydrates tends to elevate insulin, much as happens with excess cortisol, and with the same results – more of the calories end up stored as fat, and less go to everyday use. According to the theory, this can leave the body without enough energy for its metabolic needs, prompting the desire to eat more. It is not overeating which creates fat deposits, the argument goes, but the other way round.

This is the basis for the many dozens of diet books advocating a so-called ketogenic, or 'keto' diet, one based around an ultra-low carbohydrate intake and often a decidedly gung-ho attitude to ingesting fats. Acolytes have bacon for breakfast, perk themselves up with a 'bulletproof coffee', which has a lump of butter whizzed up in it, and go slightly pale if they even see a potato, let alone a slice of bread.

The keto idea has dominated diet debates in recent years, and has been enthusiastically endorsed by a string of celebrities. Does it work? The research is mixed. Quite a few studies have shown a very low carbohydrate intake can bring a relatively rapid loss of weight, although some of these have questioned the longevity of this effect. Others have raised concerns about potential side-effects, mainly based around an over-reliance on fatty proteins, including an increase in fat levels in the blood, and a higher risk of heart disease and colon cancer.

While the keto diet can and does help some people lose weight, more generally there is a definite worry about oversimplification in blaming just one food type for obesity. Human metabolism is complex, but sheer nutrient overload does appear to play a part. Yes, too much carbohydrate will be a problem. But so, most likely, will too much fat – and even too much protein. There is emerging evidence that a diet very heavy in protein can cause a rise in cortisol levels and is by no means a guaranteed escape from metabolic disorders. We now know that high bodily concentrations of something called branched-chain amino acids, which are particularly prevalent in meat and dairy products, are linked to insulin resistance. A telling example of this is the levels of type 2 diabetes and obesity in Brazil and Argentina, both countries with particularly meat-heavy diets. Such is the scale of the problem that Richard has been invited to work with Brazilian scientists to try to help them understand the metabolic processes taking place.

Brown fat v. white fat

One of the trickier areas of stress physiology when it comes to weight is the role of so-called brown fat, formally known as brown adipose tissue, or BAT. The vast bulk of fat in the human body is white adipose tissue, which is split into subcutaneous and visceral types – the latter is the fat around the belly, which brings particular health worries.

BAT is, in contrast, a tiny proportion of overall fat. While it can make up as much as 5 per cent of the weight of a newborn baby, adults often have only 50g or less, scattered at various points around the body. In fact, before the advent of infrared thermography, which allowed scientists to distinguish between brown and white fat, the common consensus was that BAT – which gets its colour from the presence of a compound which binds to iron – barely existed in adults, if at all.

We now know that in metabolic terms, BAT punches well above its weight. It plays a key role in helping the body respond to colder temperatures, with research calculating that in some situations it might be the trigger for 20 per cent of metabolic energy expended. It has also been shown that BAT can communicate with other fat tissues, despite the fact they are in different parts of the body.

> In terms of stress, the role of BAT remains uncertain. One US study found that it potentially worsens the body's inflammatory response to stress – when the scientists artificially blocked signals from the brain to brown fat deposits in mice, stress no longer caused inflammation.
>
> But at the same time, the disproportionate role of brown fat in thermogenesis, the production of heat in the body, burns a lot of calories. Slimmer people tend to have more brown fat, and there is an argument that stimulating BAT can help with weight loss. Some studies have suggested that this process can be stimulated by artificial coldness, for example a chilly shower first thing in the morning.

The carbs v. protein wars are not about to be resolved anytime soon. But from the perspective of stress, there are a couple of things to bear in mind. The first is evidence that consuming deliberately minimal amounts of carbohydrate can be perceived by the HPA axis as a threat to bodily homeostasis, especially if it involves a lower overall caloric intake than normal. This can elevate cortisol levels, potentially undoing any weight-shifting work.

Yet again, the evidence is slightly mixed. There seems to be a broad consensus that it can happen in the short term, but some studies suggest cortisol levels might then gradually return to normal – although even here, exercise appears to cause a renewed spike.

Slightly more complicated but potentially more worrying is the way that a lack of carbohydrates appears to reduce the activity of an exotic-sounding enzyme called thyroxine 5-deiodinase. As the name suggests, this is connected to the work of the thyroid gland in the throat. The gland mainly secretes the hormone thyroxine, also called T4.

This is the inactive form, and it needs thyroxine 5-deiodinase to convert it into triiodothyronine, aka T3. T3 is central to the work of the thyroid gland, which has a key role in muscle control, brain function, bone remodelling, as well as our heart and digestive functions. If thyroxine 5-deiodinase is not properly doing its work, that can lead to low levels of T3, otherwise known as hypothyroidism, meaning an under-active thyroid gland. This can cause an array of symptoms including fatigue, chronic pain, and – you guessed it – increased weight.

You might be forgiven right now for finding this chapter slightly frustrating in its lack of clear answers. In our defence, both obesity in general, and the way it relates to stress, are simply like that – no one has precisely worked out what is going on. More glibly, if we did have clear answers which definitely worked, we would currently be writing a diet book and then preparing to retire to the Maldives. But do not despair. There are things to be learned, and one of the lessons is to take an approach already seen a few times in this book: look at things from another perspective.

BMI, and whether it matters

We have talked a lot about weight and obesity without, thus far, defining what they mean. In the majority of scientific studies this involves body mass index, or BMI. As a measurement, this has existed for slightly more than fifty years, its use gradually spreading from academia to everyday life. The ubiquity of BMI is a function of simplicity: it works out whether you are overweight using the very basic means of comparing your weight with your height. BMI is your weight in kilos divided by the square of your height in metres, a calculation that can be easily done on a vast variety of websites and apps. The standard guide for the number that emerges is that, for adults, less than 18.5 is considered underweight while 18.5 to 25 is, as the NHS calculator calls it, a healthy weight. From 25 to 30 means overweight, and anything above 30 counts as obese. There are various gradations above thirty, including 'severe obesity' for figures of more than 40, but this tends to stray more into the clinical world.

BMI is very simple to work out, and it can be useful. However, it has a series of drawbacks, one fairly well known, others less so. The problem that many people know is that BMI does not distinguish between lean muscle and fat, meaning that extremely fit but bulky athletes can produce BMI numbers well above the supposedly healthy range. One recent study in medical journal *The Lancet* used the simple ruse of taking the physical details of players competing in the under-20s Six Nations rugby union tournament from squad statistics published beforehand. Of the tournament's ninety-four forwards, which includes the traditionally big men who push in a scrum, sixty-one had BMIs over 30. Officially, they were obese – a word which, for all its clinical definition, can often feel shaming and judgemental. Within that wider group there were thirty-three props, the players who lead the charge in a scrum and tend to be the biggest of all. Every single one had a BMI above 30, and for eleven of them it was above 35.

One of the less well-known issues with BMI is that while many people understand that the problems begin above a figure of 25, they might not know that this metric was devised entirely by studies involving men, meaning there is some debate about how useful such a broad gauge is for women in any case. It was also based almost entirely on research among people of European heritage. This is a particularly important point for people of South Asian backgrounds, given that research suggests they can be susceptible to health problems, particularly type 2 diabetes, at lower BMI readings. There are various theories as to why this is the case, including the apparent tendency of people of South Asian heritage to store fat more around their organs rather than just beneath their skin. The World Health Organization therefore recommends that for people of South Asian origin, the tipping point for being overweight should be seen as 23 rather than 25, with obesity starting at 27.5.

*

Most crucial of all for BMI, and even less well known, is something particularly relevant for stress: when it comes to long-term health,

BMI might not be a useful measure at all. Instead, a mass of new research suggests that waist size could be a better gauge. Much as BMI is a proxy for overall potential obesity, waist size serves as a stand-in for the build-up of abdominal fat associated with high cortisol, and thus the metabolic and other problems which come from it.

In the simplest terms, the medical advice says that whatever your height or your BMI, if you are a man you should be worried if your waist circumference is more than 37 inches (94cm), while for women it's 31.5 inches (80cm). Much above this – 40 inches (101.5cm) for men and 34.5 inches (87.5cm) for women – and NHS guidance suggests you see a doctor. A slightly more sophisticated model is waist-to-height ratio. Here, a figure of 0.4 to 0.49 is seen as healthy, with 0.5 and above bringing health risks, all the more so above 0.6.

Most people know their waist size, but mainly for buying clothes. Medically, it doesn't get nearly as much attention as BMI. This is a shame for a series of reasons, particularly when it comes to people for whom worries about weight might be connected to stress. The first issue is that stomach-based fat, as we saw above, is often a specific consequence of chronic stress. A bigger waist is also linked to health issues themselves made worse by stress, such as insulin resistance. Additionally, as we have also seen, people with an apple-type body appear to react more sensitively to cortisol.

The final reason to consider waist size is notably more positive: unlike BMI, it is something that does not seem virtually impossible to reduce. A whole mass of studies have shown that exercise, particularly a combination of aerobic and weight-bearing exertion, if maintained over a period, tends to have a notably beneficial impact on your waistline. One recent meta-study, in which scientists crunched the data from twenty-five existing trials, found an average reduction in waist circumference of 3.2cm for aerobic activity alone.[13] This is perhaps the biggest disadvantage of the endless focus on BMI, or on the raw numbers of bodily weight. It is not uncommon for people to become considerably more active, then find that their BMI is resolutely unchanged and give up on their new regime as they think it's not doing them any good. Nothing could be further from the truth. More or less any amount of extra movement, in more or less any circumstance, makes you healthier.

This is something we delve into in greater detail in Chapter 10, but as a message it is particularly pertinent when it comes to the types of ailments made worse by stress, notably insulin resistance, which is hugely responsive to physical movement. Focusing on waist size rather than BMI can help make it seem real.

This brings us back to Ellie. Ellie still prefers not to know what she weighs, and she is still in psychotherapy, thinking about her body image issues. She still looks at other people's toned physiques on social media more than she would like to. But she joined a gym, and four months later, after regular aerobic classes and weight-based exercises – she was advised to avoid too many high-intensity sessions – her cortisol levels are slightly lower. Her blood glucose has fallen only marginally, but this is a measure which tends to be hard to shift, even when insulin begins to work better. More tests are needed, but the signs are that Ellie is no longer on a likely trajectory towards insulin resistance. As well as being averse to scales, she is not especially keen on measuring her waist, but the general signs are good. 'There's definitely something happening,' she says. 'My clothes just seem to hang on me better.'

And what of Andrej? As an elite footballer in a European league, he is already surrounded by a raft of experts and has no need for a UK-based clinic – his story was recounted to Richard by a professional contact. He worked hard with his team's doctors and physiotherapists to rebuild the muscle he had lost. He also discussed his body-image worries with a sports psychologist. The success of this regime can be seen via very obvious metrics which are not translatable to the everyday world, such as the number of minutes played and goals scored. He is now back in the team and playing well. Defenders once again seem to bounce off him. He is still loved by the fans.

This is a complex and nuanced area, even by the standards of stress science, not to mention one that is even more subject to stigma and guilt. But equally, it is something that cannot be ignored. All stress, if sufficiently intense and prolonged, carries some risks to our health. But when it is combined with a gain in weight, particularly in certain parts of the body, this effect is magnified. And much of the risks come from that most ubiquitous of modern medical conditions, the subject of our next chapter: type 2 diabetes.

CHAPTER 7

The Tidal Wave of Illness: Stress and Diabetes

The medical condition which presents probably the biggest single threat to the viability of universal healthcare systems across the globe is in many ways so subtle, so low-key, that around half of the people who have it don't yet know this. Many millions more are on the path towards developing it in the future. This is a tidal wave of illness, and it is breaking out over the globe almost in silence. This is type 2 diabetes – and, as we are about to see, it is very often connected to stress.

How many people actually have type 2 diabetes? No one is even approximately sure. The best estimates put it somewhere north of 500 million people worldwide, around 240 million of whom have not yet had the condition diagnosed. Within a decade or so, somewhere close to 800 million could be affected.[1]

One thing is certain: its incidence is increasing at pace, and on several new fronts at once. Previously known as an ailment of the middle-aged and middle class, often in wealthier nations, the bulk of the rise in type 2 diabetes cases is coming from what are officially known as low-to-middle-income countries. The ten places with the highest per-capita prevalence of type 2 diabetes include the US, Japan and Italy, but also India, China, Indonesia and Bangladesh. Additionally, a condition once known as 'adult-onset diabetes', to distinguish it from type 1 diabetes, is increasingly being seen in young people. Until a few decades ago it barely existed in anyone below their thirties, even forties. Now it is being regularly spotted in adolescents, and increasingly often in children.[2]

Estimating the cost of all this in healthcare terms is necessarily approximate, but some put it at close to, if not already past, US$1 trillion globally. Many people with type 2 diabetes are put on a regime of several drugs which could well be needed for the rest of their lives. Numerous doctors in the UK's NHS warn that with the current rate of growth of this and other chronic health conditions, free universal healthcare will soon become unsustainable.

This is largely a disease of lifestyle, albeit with some apparent genetic input into your propensity to develop it. The biggest triggers include excess weight, particularly fat around the organs, and a lack of physical activity, with the latter seen as particularly relevant for younger people.

> ## What is type 2 diabetes?
>
> Diabetes is a condition in which the body is unable to properly process blood sugars in response to insulin, the hormone which does this job, not functioning properly. In type 1 diabetes, an autoimmune disease generally diagnosed when people are young, the body simply doesn't produce insulin.
>
> In the type 2 version, insulin is produced, but for what can be a variety of reasons it does not perform its function as well as it should. Type 2 more often emerges in later adulthood, and is closely linked to lifestyle factors such as weight and long-term physical inactivity.

However, stress can play a central role. If chronic stress is, in physiological terms, bodily homeostasis knocked off-balance, then so-called metabolic conditions like type 2 diabetes can often be an eventual end point for all this. Much as you could never properly look at stress without thinking about the way repeated cortisol spikes affect the way we process blood sugars, trying to tackle type 2 diabetes without considering stress would be to see just half the picture.

One of the most alarming things about type 2 diabetes is that the standard diagnostic test, based on blood sugar levels, often fails to catch it early enough. The starting point of the condition is insulin resistance, where the body fails to respond properly to the hormone and so increases how much it secretes. However, the extra insulin tends to keep blood sugar levels appearing normal for a period, until the insulin secretion system in the pancreas becomes, in effect, exhausted by this endless feedback loop. Elevated insulin, formally known as hyperinsulinemia, is often a path towards diabetes. But by the time things are bad enough for it to be diagnosed, the bodily damage might have already started. Discovering all this before the problems mount up can be difficult.

Take the example of Yusuf, a 46-year-old media executive; he was another apparent metabolic puzzle to arrive at the clinic. His BMI was 28, above the healthy guideline of 25, if not vastly so. His reading for visceral fat, the type that sits on the belly and around the organs, was slightly higher than ideal. Much of this might be normal for someone of his age, but Yusuf was perturbed: he was eating well and exercised regularly. He did not understand why he did not weigh less.

Tests detected blood glucose levels within normal parameters, but also slightly elevated cortisol. Was the higher-than-normal cortisol – likely to be the product of a job Yusuf fully admitted was hectic, along with the pressure of helping to care for his elderly parents – the end of the matter? Or could it be indicating insulin resistance?

Many clinics claim to measure not just full diabetes but also prediabetes, through blood glucose measurements including one called the HbA1c test, which gives an average reading for the last three months. This is impressive, but again, if extra surges of insulin are keeping sugar levels within the normal range, then the HbA1c readings might mask the real situation. A gold-standard test for insulin sensitivity does exist, but it is fairly cumbersome and rarely seen outside academic laboratories. Known slightly alarmingly as the insulin clamp, it doesn't involve any hefty pieces of metal pinning the patient's arm to a bed. The clamp in this case refers to the way insulin and glucose are infused intravenously, with the amount of insulin in the person's blood kept elevated but steady, with a variable amount of glucose used to keep the person's blood glucose level 'clamped' at a set level. If minimal glucose is required to maintain this level, it indicates that insulin is not operating effectively. If their system is working well, they are insulin-sensitive. If not, they are showing signs of insulin resistance.

Short of getting Yusuf enrolled in a university study, this wasn't possible. There was something of a workaround, however. If you test a person's so-called fasting blood glucose levels, when they have not eaten for twelve hours or so, and also test their fasting insulin levels, the readings can be compared to give a score on something called, a bit clunkily, the homeostasis model assessment of insulin resistance, often shortened to HOMA-IR. This has only recently moved from research work to use in clinics, and the results it produces are only a broad guide. A figure of 1.5 or greater is generally seen as putting someone into insulin resistance, with anything above 3 seen as type 2 diabetes — with the caveat that readings can vary between different population groups. Yusuf's score was 1.8.

What did this mean? Within some bounds of doubt, he was most likely to be prediabetic or approaching that state, and to continue on the same metabolic path could see him become fully diabetic. Also, given his otherwise healthy lifestyle, it appeared that stress could well be a factor, with a bit of heredity added in.

There was another factor to consider: ethnicity. This was potentially significant in two ways. The first, as already mentioned, is that studies show people from minority ethnic backgrounds tend to experience above-average levels of stress. There is even UK-specific research indicating that this is the case for people of South Asian heritage, and those who are Muslim, both directly relevant to Yusuf. But also, there is something to consider when it comes to the impacts of stress. Britons of South Asian descent are six times more likely to have type 2 diabetes than the population as a whole. This is partly related to diet and lifestyle, but also appears to be a factor of genetics and the way people from this ethnicity metabolize fats. Scientists don't yet fully understand the way this works, but the risks are very real, and this meant Yusuf's score was all the more likely to be a sign of insulin resistance.

How could stress affect this? We will get into the full science a bit further on, but to an extent, it is almost the job description for stress hormones. As we saw in previous chapters, when the alarm response kicks in, a rush of cortisol flowing through the body prompts the release of energy from short-term stores of glucose, immediately raising blood sugar levels to provide energy to deal with a threat. This is a perfectly sensible response in evolutionary terms, but when repeated endlessly it gives the pancreas the job of producing more and more insulin to get blood sugar levels back to normal. The eventual result is often that the body's tissues become gradually less responsive to insulin. This was the point where Yusuf seemed to have found himself.

In some ways, even this was not a completely satisfactory answer. Yusuf's body was reacting badly to circumstances which were not necessarily within his control. The way to get to grips with it was not obvious. But it was an answer of sorts, yet one denied to the great majority of people who, unlike Yusuf, cannot afford to pay for their own tests at a private clinic.

Most people probably know at least someone who lives with type 2 diabetes. And yet it remains in part a mystery, especially the interaction with stress. This is in many ways nothing new. Since the very existence of medicine itself, diabetes has often been a condition that provides more questions than answers.

The long sorrow

In what is believed to be the earliest-ever written medical reference to diabetes of any sort, Sushrata, a Hindu surgeon who practised in northern India as early as the sixth century BC, described a phenomenon in which some patients had the curious symptom of urine that tasted sweet and would attract ants. He said the ailment tended to run in families and was most common in well-off people who were overweight and indolent, even going so far as to link it to their high consumption of food like sweets and rice.

Aside from the uncannily accurate description of the likely lifestyles of people at risk of developing type 2 diabetes, the giveaway is the reference to the sweetness of urine. In a healthy body, homeostasis keeps the amount of glucose in your blood at around 4–5.5 millimoles per litre when you have not eaten for some hours, a level maintained by insulin. However, if that process is not working properly and blood glucose rises, your kidneys cannot reabsorb it so the excess sugars are removed in urine. In the many centuries before the advent of blood glucose tests, doctors would often taste urine to detect diabetes.

Sushrata – who, it should be noted, is believed by many historians to have been a series of authors contributing over time to the same text – also distinguished between two apparently different groups affected by what he (or they) called *madhumeha*, a term meaning 'honey urine'. One was the high-living, overweight, middle-aged patients, but there were also those who developed the malady when young and slim. There are, of course, two main types of diabetes, and while they have a central point in common – a dysfunction of insulin and the resultant inability to process blood sugar – they are different afflictions.

Type 1 diabetes is an auto-immune condition in which the body's immune system attacks the beta cells in the pancreas which produce insulin. It can be diagnosed in adulthood but it more usually emerges in childhood or adolescence. It is much less common than its type 2 neighbour, with perhaps 1 in 1,000 people having it. Some research suggests slightly more cases of type 1 are being diagnosed, and as well as a hereditary element, research has shown it can also have environmental triggers including diet, obesity and exposure to certain viruses. Intriguingly, other studies have indicated that early-life experiences, including parental stress, can increase a child's propensity to develop the condition. There is also a correlation between family poverty and type 1 diabetes, including relative poverty in an otherwise wealthy nation.

Type 2, as we have already seen, is more directly associated with lifestyle (and also with poverty), and is increasing in prevalence all the time. A bit confusingly, there is also a form of diabetes which is something of a cross between the two. Officially called latent autoimmune diabetes in adults, or type 1.5, like type 2 it is generally diagnosed in adults and is slow-developing, but it is an auto-immune condition like type 1, and most people who develop it require treatment with insulin at some point.

Thomas Wolsey: Cardinal, royal confidant – and diabetic?

Trying to retrospectively diagnose figures from history with type 2 diabetes is a necessarily approximate exercise, but even though he lived over 500 years ago, one of the most likely candidates appears to be Thomas Wolsey.

An extraordinary figure of his era, who rose from deeply humble origins – born in Ipswich, his father is believed to have been a butcher – Wolsey became a cardinal in the Catholic church as well as Lord Chancellor, in effect chief adviser to Henry VIII. In the latter role he spent nearly fifteen years effectively running many affairs of state, including overseas relations.

Catholic clergy might be seen as generally ascetic and moderate in their appetites. Even setting aside the fact that Wolsey fathered two children, he was not in that mould. Very obviously corpulent in the most famous painting of him, contemporary accounts of banquets he hosted give some idea as to why he might have been susceptible to the condition.

One such feast included courses of boar, venison, swan, peacock and lobster, generally served with rich sauces and followed by sugary

> desserts. There was also a liberal ingestion of butter, something suggested by doctors of the time as a healthy way to begin a meal. Wolsey was later reported to have developed serious eye troubles, a sign of poorly-managed diabetes. The only treatments on offer were bleeding or purging, aimed at restoring the balance of bodily humors, the sixteenth century's version of homeostasis.
>
> As even non-history buffs generally know, Henry VIII's links with the Catholic church did not end well. Wolsey was arrested in 1530 and accused of treason. Perhaps luckily for him, on his way from York to London to stand trial, the 59-year-old cardinal died after succumbing – according to some historians – to a diabetic coma.

Finally, there is gestational diabetes, which affects some women in pregnancy when they cannot produce enough insulin amid everything else that is going on in their bodies. This is not type 2, and it ceases when the baby is born. However, it does have some parallels in that a risk factor can be the mother's weight, and the fact that women who develop it are more likely to get type 2 diabetes later in life – although neither is necessarily the case.

All the types have a very obvious common factor: insulin. The long medical history of attempts to treat diabetes was, in effect, a hunt for insulin, which has a case for being the single most impactful hormone in our body, as discovered by Yusuf. Its eventual isolation in 1921, and then its production as a treatment for type 1 diabetes, was one of the greatest medical breakthroughs of that century, in part as this also helped scientists better comprehend type 2.

It was not a quick process. One of the first scientists to understand diabetes rather than simply describe it was Thomas Willis, a celebrated English anatomist of the seventeenth century, even if he did incorrectly ascribe it as a disorder of the blood. However, he also very perceptively identified what we now know are two major factors in the genesis of type 2 diabetes: indulgent living and mental distress. In his 1679 book *Pharmaceutice rationalis, sive diatriba de medicamentorum operationibus in humano corpore*, Latin for *Rational Medicine, or An Exercitation of the Operations of Medicine in the Human Body*, Willis attributed the condition not only to 'immoderate drinking of cider, beer and sharp wines' but also to extended sadness, or, as he eloquently termed it, 'the long sorrow'.[3]

Willis noted the increased urine production of diabetic patients, memorably describing the condition as 'the pissing evil'. He also rediscovered – or arguably discovered, given Sushrata's works were unknown to him – the sweet taste of diabetic urine, adding to diabetes the word *mellitis*, Latin for honeyed or sweet, a coda which remains in its formal name today. He was, however, unable to give an explanation for the taste. This fell to another English physician and diabetes pioneer, Matthew Dobson, who worked it out a century later by boiling down the urine of someone with diabetes and finding it left behind a sugar-like residue.

One of the first major breakthroughs into understanding how sugars are actually processed in the body – and what would be key to the condition – came thanks to the work of a familiar name: Claude Bernard, the inventor of the idea of the *milieu intérieur*, who we heard about at length in Chapter 4. In 1857, twenty-one years before he came up with his unifying theory, Bernard explained to a scientific lecture in Paris the fruits of his long and often brutal experiments on a series of dogs. First he had disproved his initial theory that bodily sugars were processed in the lungs by injecting grape sugar into the jugular vein of a dog and immediately extracting blood from its carotid artery. The blood, which biologically had to have passed through the lungs, still contained significant amounts of sugar.[4]

After feeding other dogs various diets and immediately killing them, he worked out that blood sugars did not always come directly from food. This mass of dissections did, however, find that every animal's liver contained a starchy fluid which he called glycogen, a form of glucose that can be stored and used for bodily energy, and which is broken down under the impact of cortisol.

Although Bernard incorrectly concluded that excess glycogen in the liver is the cause of diabetes – in fact, it is a potential complication of the condition – this was a major advance. It came, however, at some apparent personal cost. Much as the anti-vivisection movement taking shape in England in the second half of the nineteenth century was mainly led by women, so it was in France, and among the French activists was Marie-Françoise Bernard, better known as Fanny, who happened to be Bernard's wife. While historians cannot be sure that Fanny's dislike of her husband's endless experiments on dogs was the reason behind their formal separation in 1870 – no small matter for a respectable Catholic couple in that era – Fanny and her two daughters went on to set up a shelter for stray dogs and cats, which gives a fairly clear sign of her views. Bernard vigorously defended his animal experiments, and when it came to a treatment for diabetes, most scientists of the time backed him. For some people, they argued, this was a matter of life and death.

More than a century after insulin was identified and isolated, and now that type 1 diabetics can maintain their blood sugar using insulin pens or a continually-monitored feed from a pump, it can be difficult to understand how devastating the disease was before this point, both for patients and their families. For a very long time the general prognosis was that people who started to show symptoms simply would not live much longer. Even around the start of the twentieth century, a pioneering diabetes expert who knew as much about the condition as anyone said that the average life expectancy of a ten-year-old diagnosed with type 1 was just over a year, while aged thirty it was about four years.

This was Elliott Joslin, whose diabetes foundation, established in Boston in the US in 1898, is still a leading research centre into the condition. Joslin's medical career spanned either side of the insulin revolution. Before it was isolated and used, more or less the only way he could treat people with type 1 diabetes was by maintaining them in a sort of perpetual half-life where they subsisted – usually bed-bound and sometimes barely strong enough to move – on tiny amounts of food, particularly lacking in carbohydrates.

Joslin had what was described as a 'prize patient', a seventeen-year-old girl, who was 5 feet tall. She weighed 25kg, roughly the same as an average eight- or nine-year-old girl today. Another of his patients, a fifteen-year-old girl, lived on a daily diet of 30g of fat, 25g of protein, and precisely 6g of carbohydrates. The latter is roughly equivalent to a tenth of a standard serving of pasta in a single meal.[5]

Joslin was challenged on his methods, and himself openly wondered if it might be better to allow his patients a normal diet and a happier, if shorter, life. The one reason he kept on with such a regime was the hope that a treatment could arrive at any time.

By this point scientists knew the vital substance was secreted from the pancreas, located in the abdomen, after a German physiologist called Oskar Minkowski found that removing the organ from dogs caused them to become diabetic. A whole series of researchers raced to close in on the mystery, a battle so hard-fought that there are even two competing claims to have come up with the name 'insulin', from a British scientist and a Belgian one in the first decade of the twentieth century.

The team who built on all these efforts to finally produce medically useable insulin was a Canadian-Scottish-American co-production which, as is often the case with such scientific triumphs, gained the plaudits in part by being in the right place at the right time – and then proceeded to squabble bitterly over the credit. At the centre was Frederick Banting, a young orthopaedic surgeon at Toronto University who only became interested in diabetes research after being obliged to read about carbohydrate metabolism, a subject he was no expert on, for a student lecture he was due to deliver. By this point a series of other researchers had already tried to use pancreatic extracts to treat diabetes, but no one had found a way to separate out what came from the islets of Langerhans, the exotically-named pancreatic element which includes insulin-producing beta cells. Banting hit upon a possible way to do this, by closing the pancreatic ducts, which carry digestive secretions. The effect of this was that the main part of the pancreas degenerated, while the islets of Langerhans were unaffected.

Banting, who was somewhat hapless when it came to laboratory work, asked for the help of John Macleod, a more experienced Scottish academic at the university, who had ended up in Canada via the US. Somewhat sceptical about Banting's mission, Macleod lent him a disused laboratory and the assistance of two students. The students tossed a coin to see who would be enlisted, and the US-born Charles Best either won or lost, depending on your view.

Despite Macleod's doubts, Banting's idea worked. He and Best managed to produce an extract from the endocrine part of a dog's pancreas, which was then injected into another dog whose own pancreas had been removed. The latter animal's blood sugar levels started to fall. The successful experiment was repeated, and also worked using extracts from calf pancreases. On 11 January 1922, the first human patient to receive artificially extracted insulin was injected in the buttock at Toronto General Hospital with what one of the ward doctors described as '15cc of brown muck'. Leonard Thompson was fourteen, severely underweight and kept drifting into a diabetic coma, so his parents believed he had nothing to lose. As it turned out, the first jab had not been very well prepared, and while it caused his blood sugar levels to fall, it also led to a nasty allergic abscess. With the assistance of James Collip, a biochemist at the university who had provided vital help in purifying Banting and Macleod's substances, a better version was prepared. Twelve days later, Thompson received a second injection. This worked, with no unpleasant side effects. The teenager was in remission. Regular insulin injections saw him live until twenty-seven, when he was killed by pneumonia, very possibly a result of his earlier struggles with diabetes.

A March 1922 edition of the *Canadian Medical Association Journal* reported the team's successful trials on seven patients, who not only saw lower blood sugar readings but appeared able to consume carbohydrates normally, regaining their vigour. This was little short of a miracle cure. Insulin was, as one newspaper called it shortly afterwards, 'a force of magical activity'.[6]

Unsurprisingly, the discovery caught the attention of the Nobel Prize committee for Medicine. More contentiously, they awarded it in 1923 just to Banting and Macleod, ignoring the roles of Best and Collip. Banting shared his prize money with Best, and Macleod with Collip, but the omission caused years of subsequent acrimony within the group, which only ended when Banting was killed in an air crash in 1941.

A very curious side note to this quarrelling is that there is a case to be made for a completely different researcher having beaten them to it by more than twenty years. This was Eugène Gley, a French endocrinologist who had discovered the small parathyroid glands in the neck during the 1880s. He then spent the next decade developing a pancreatic extract which he found improved diabetic symptoms in dogs, and which in later experiments demonstrated was connected to the islets of Langerhans.

Any modern researcher would rush their findings to a journal, as Banting did in 1922. Gley, however, wrote them down and placed this in a sealed envelope which he left with the *Société de Biologie* in Paris, with strict instructions that it should not be opened unless he said so. The contents were read only in 1922, after Banting and his colleagues had announced their discovery and claimed the plaudits. Such modesty appears baffling, but the practice was not unknown among scientists of the period if they felt their research needed gaps filled in by others. Gley's retrospective coup won little attention, and nearly a century after his death he is only remembered in medical circles. Banting, in contrast, was feted from the moment the news of the discovery was announced, especially after he was awarded a patent for insulin and immediately sold it for $1 to Toronto University, who licensed the miracle cure without cost to overseas non-profit groups. By early 1923 insulin was being mass-produced and saving lives around the world. Banting's birthday, 14 November, is still marked as World Diabetes Day.

The modern pandemic

Between 1875 and 1895, the Manchester Royal Infirmary, the English city's main public hospital, admitted precisely 272 people with diabetes, almost 0.1 per cent of the 27,721 in-patients it received over those two decades. Now part of the wider Manchester University NHS Foundation Trust, the modern Royal Infirmary has an entire diabetes centre, staffed by specialist doctors, nurses and dietitians, with separate sections for research and education, a full-time admissions service for people with diabetes and a range of outpatients clinics for problems involving people's feet, joints and kidneys, and one dedicated to young people.

NHS-wide statistics say that while around 1 in 17 of the population as a whole has diabetes of any type, among all patients admitted to hospitals it is about one in six.[7] The Royal Infirmary has just over 1,700 beds, meaning that on average, 280 of them contain someone with diabetes – amounting to slightly more diabetic patients in a single day than the Victorian hospital saw over twenty years.

There are a few caveats. The most obvious is that in the pre-NHS era, many fewer people sought hospital treatment, not least as you had to pay for it. Additionally, almost all Victorians with type 2 diabetes would have been fairly well off and thus not very likely to go to a public hospital. But the wider point stands: societally, diabetes is no longer the same disease.

Type 1 diabetes continues to be diagnosed at relatively low levels, and it is a serious condition, but it is one that can be maintained and lived with if managed well, thanks to Frederick Banting and his co-researchers. Type 2 diabetes is nothing new, as shown by Sushruta. It has, however, exploded in prevalence. As mentioned earlier, two of the major factors in this are obesity and physical inactivity. Both are, again, nothing new, simply much more widespread. A diet of calorically rich foods and a lifestyle in which you barely walk any distance is no longer the preserve of the very rich. In many countries, it is the default, and something which now tends to be more likely if you are poorer.

We dealt briefly with the factors behind obesogenic environments in the previous chapter, while the reasons that everyday physical movement has all but disappeared for many people are even more complex. But where does stress come into the picture? How important is it? And finally – of particular relevance to people like Yusuf – how is it able to shape your metabolic destiny even if you eat a healthy diet and move regularly? As ever with the fundamentally logical and yet very complicated world of the human metabolic system, there is a short answer and a longer one, and tacked to the end of the longer one are a series of questions for which we don't as yet have all the information.

The short answer is that the hormonal activity set in place by the stress response – a rapid uptake in quick-release glycogen from the liver – turns out to be a near-perfect bodily recipe for gradual insulin resistance if repeated too often. This is especially the case when you add in another frequent effect of cortisol, which is for it to play havoc with the breakdown of bodily fats. The surprise is less that chronically stressed people often succumb to insulin resistance than the fact that some escape this. Metabolic turmoil is arguably the norm.

The longer answer is more technical, if not necessarily much more complicated. It begins with the pancreas. This has two parts: a so-called exocrine section, about 85 per cent of the total mass, which secretes digestive enzymes; and the endocrine pancreas, aka the islets of Langerhans, which are responsible for producing insulin.

These received their evocative name because, firstly, they are scattered around the wider organ, much like islands in an ocean, and then because of Paul Langerhans, the German scientist who spotted this, in 1868. Langerhans was an extraordinarily energetic and gifted researcher whose hand-drawings of the islets, based on what he saw through a very basic microscope, look almost identical to modern digital images. Langerhans also made separate discoveries about the immune system and, after tuberculosis obliged him to relocate to the sunny Portuguese island of Madeira, became a noted zoologist, all before dying aged just forty.

Strictly speaking, although insulin production is the islets' biggest role, it's not their only one. While up to 80 per cent of the islets' mass comprises beta cells, which secrete insulin, there are also alpha, delta and epsilon cells that are responsible for, respectively: glucagon, a hormone which increases blood sugar levels, the opposite to insulin; somatostatin, a peptide hormone which has a sort of general supervisory role in the endocrine system, turning secretions off and on; and finally ghrelin, a hormone linked to the desire to eat.

Insulin has the relatively straightforward but biologically vital job of controlling blood glucose homeostasis, which it does by sorting out the transport of intracellular glucose to the bits of the body that use or store it: the liver, skeletal muscle and fat cells. It does this by stimulating the work of glucose transporter proteins, notably glucose transporter 4, or GLUT-4, the one we heard about in Chapter 4 which clears glucose from the blood by allowing it to move into skeletal muscle or fat cells. There are other versions with which insulin interacts, including GLUT-1, which is most abundant in heart muscle but also works in fat, and GLUT-13, which is particularly important in the brain.

The road towards type 2 diabetes can come in a variety of often interconnected ways. The pancreas might not produce enough insulin or bodily tissues might not respond to insulin, leading to insulin resistance. Intriguingly, not only do we not yet fully understand how the path from insulin resistance to type 2 diabetes happens, but it can take place very differently in different people, in part a function of genetics – for example, people of Greenlandic Inuit heritage who have a genetic mutation known as TBC1D4 can be highly insulin resistant while not showing hyperinsulinemia, elevated insulin levels.[8]

What is known, however, is that an eventual shortage of insulin happens because of a reduction in the number of beta cells, sometimes in combination with an increase in alpha cells, which do the opposite job. How does this happen? Because, to simplify things just slightly, beta cells don't thrive in repeated conditions of high glucose levels and exposure to more fats in the blood. And that is just what cortisol supplies.

A raft of studies have shown that chronic exposure to higher amounts of so-called free fatty acids can cause beta cells to function less well. They can also be irreversibly damaged by persistently high blood sugar levels, a state known as glucotoxicity.

This whole process is still just partly understood, and the addition of stress makes it all the more complicated. Not all cells respond to cortisol in the same way. Scientists are still a distance from being able to follow the actions of the human body's 538 so-called kinases, protein enzymes which, in effect, pass instructions to cells and influence what they do. Researchers have, thus far, identified around 7,000 of their specific interactions, leaving a mere 227,000 or so to be deciphered. Kinase-targeting drugs are a hugely exciting new frontier for clinical medicine, with applications for cancer as well as diabetes. Thus far, however, there has been regulatory approval for drugs aimed at just 22 kinases, little more than 4 per cent of the total. These are very early days.

It is not even known whether the failure of beta cells is the trigger for the silent and internal metabolic battle that leads towards type 2 diabetes, or if this failure is itself caused by an earlier process. Adding to the complications, insulin resistance can happen in two ways, which often interlink. One, known as peripheral insulin resistance, is where the reduced impact of insulin leads to less uptake of blood sugars in the parts of the body that normally do this – skeletal muscle, fat tissues and the liver. This can also prompt the release of more free fatty acids into the blood, something which in turn further inhibits the effectiveness of insulin.

The other is central, or hepatic, insulin resistance. This happens when the liver starts to produce more glucose than the body needs, knocking blood sugar homeostasis even further off-course. The role of the liver in whole-body metabolism is still being uncovered, but it is seen as central to this process.

The inescapable burden

The landmark *Whitehall Two* study, which we discussed earlier in the book, helped to definitively show that stress is not a product of high status and seniority, but more often than not the opposite. But that was not its only lesson. Generally, once researchers have gathered a mass cohort of people and observed them over time, more conclusions inevitably emerge. And so it was after the 10,000 or so UK civil servants had periodically answered questions and underwent medical checks for *Whitehall Two*.

Later analysis found that stress at work made people much more likely to develop metabolic disorders like type 2 diabetes, and that these were notably more prevalent among officials in lower-grade roles. When the data was adjusted to allow for people's age and job seniority, those who reported three or more periods of what they saw as chronic work stress were over twice as likely to have bodily markers indicating a path towards type 2 diabetes than those who said they had faced none.[9]

Later studies have come to very similar conclusions. Danish research which spent a decade looking at 7,000-plus men and women with the extremely broad age range of 20 to 93 found that those who said they were stressed – this time whether at home or work – were twice as likely to develop diabetes.[10]

A separate and even longer-term study, tracking over 7,000 Swedes, men only this time, for a Herculean thirty-five-year period, found that, after adjusting for age and other medical conditions, those with long-term stress were notably more likely to be diagnosed with diabetes. This did not mean that those without stress were immune. Overall, 31 per cent of this group developed diabetes, but that was compared with 43 per cent of the chronically stressed.

Factors like weight and inactivity play a major role; stress just makes things even worse.[11]

Significantly, only people who said they were permanently stressed saw this increased likelihood. The rate of diabetes among those who occasionally experienced stress was almost exactly the same as the professedly never-stressed. The length of time and lack of let-up seems to be what ultimately wears down metabolic homeostasis.

A crucial point to also note is that, as we saw in the last chapter with the effect of stress on weight, there is a good deal of circularity. To take one example: in addition to those studies showing that stressed people are more likely to develop type 2 diabetes, other research shows that people who already have diabetes tend to be more stressed than average, and to also show greater propensities to depression and anger. In part this will be because of residual pre-diagnosis characteristics. But simply having diabetes is known to be a stressor, involving everything from an often complex drug regime to worries about diet and potential future complications.

Similarly, many of the lifestyle behaviours that worsen metabolic disorders are closely linked to long-term stress, not least being overweight or obese. As we saw in the last chapter, as well as changing the way the body processes fats, stress often makes someone gravitate towards higher-calorie and less nutritious foods. Other studies have shown that if you are chronically stressed you are more likely to be physically inactive and to sit down for long periods, both major risks for type 2 diabetes.

As if all this was not enough of a worry, research has shown that a generalized tendency towards the sorts of bodily markers indicating future type 2 diabetes – fat around the abdomen, high fasting blood sugar and elevated fats in the blood – seems to also increase the risk of developing some cancers, as well as heart disease. It is such a broad picture that a cluster of these signs is often just labelled as 'metabolic syndrome', or more ominously, 'Syndrome X'.

This broad phenomenon is sometimes assessed using the slightly wider measure of allostatic load, as seen in Chapter 4. Here, the idea of a bodily system chronically lacking homeostasis is examined using ten measures, including blood sugar and cholesterol levels, waist-to-hip ratio, blood pressure, and the prevalence of stress hormones including cortisol and adrenaline. It also measures levels of dehydroepiandrosterone sulfate, a sex hormone present in men and women and produced by the adrenal glands. Elevated levels of this, usually shortened to DHEA sulfate, are often a sign of stress.

This is complicated and time-consuming stuff, and not easy within the necessarily limited medical bandwidth of a system like the NHS. The UK's health service does offer a check-up for the middle-aged which focuses heavily on type 2 diabetes as well as heart disease. However, beyond height, weight, blood pressure and cholesterol, it mainly considers risk factors like family health history and activity levels. It can provide warnings, but not an early diagnosis.

Yusuf, in contrast, had at least part of an answer, if one that did not seem to offer much of a way forward. He was living a healthy lifestyle yet was potentially on the path to diabetes. The insulin resistance score of 1.8 had spooked him. What could he do next? In a pattern you might by now recognize from our earlier case histories, the solution was not a lifestyle revolution, or a single, dramatic step, or even a checklist of things to do. It was a series of tweaks, modifications and gradual realizations, some of which turned out to be unexpected.

The starting point was stress. Yusuf was fortunate enough to be sufficiently senior in his job that he could delegate certain tasks; and, as is often the case, the moment he did this he realized that at least part of his workload was less a product of necessity than a desire to feel indispensable. As the eldest sibling, he had also taken on the bulk of the responsibility over the welfare of his parents, again on an assumption that no one else could or would do it. But his brother and sister were happy to contribute more, giving Yusuf even more time with his immediate family.

Another element was a surprise to Yusuf, if less so to a healthcare profession well versed in the maxim that people almost inevitably underestimate how much they eat and overestimate how much they move. A food-and-exercise diary showed that while Yusuf's meals at home were largely healthy, a work-related regime of snacks and client dinners meant his daily food intake averaged around 2,800 calories, 300 calories above the NHS recommendation for men. Similarly, his recollection of his exercise patterns appeared to be based more on his situation a couple of years earlier, when he had been training for a half-marathon. Post-diary, his diet featured fewer pastries and meals doused in Thomas Wolsey-style rich sauces, and his week now included more time spent running. He also started using a sit-stand desk at work to avoid very long periods sitting down.

Six months later, Yusuf's homeostasis model assessment of insulin resistance score was 1.5, still slightly above the ideal but on the right trajectory.

There was one other change. After learning his original test score, and that not everyone has the same bodily reaction to stress hormones, Yusuf was prompted to do something he had considered anyway: he began weekly psychotherapy. In particular, he wanted to explore things which might contribute to a cortisol-reactive disposition. This proved a revelation, if not always a completely comfortable one. Talking at length about his childhood, Yusuf began to understand the way he had always shouldered responsibility, from a very young age. Six years older than his sister and with parents who worked long hours running their own small business, he often walked her to and from school, even making her evening meal and sometimes putting her to bed. Talking about his parents, he also began to understand how stressed they had been, and often mentally absent, as far back as he could remember.

Yusuf's is just one case history. As with everything connected to stress, no two people will be the same. A propensity to type 2 diabetes can be the product of numerous factors, particularly diet, weight and activity levels, although all these can also be tied in to stress.

There is, however, one stress-connected physical consequence that is generally less well known, and which is particularly weighed down by cultural assumptions, as well as, all too often, by shame and stigma. This is infertility. Yet again, it is a story of many different parts.

CHAPTER 8

The Delicate Balance: How Stress Can Affect Fertility

It can be a desperately difficult and often isolating process, trying again and again to conceive a child in a world where, it sometimes feels, almost everyone else is pregnant or holding a baby. However little comfort it might be, this is not actually the case: infertility is an increasingly significant problem. And it seems beyond any doubt that stress, among many factors, is playing a part.

Probably the most definitive statistics for infertility as a general phenomenon came a few years ago with data collated by something called the Global Burden of Disease, a vast and ongoing international project which gathers health information on all sorts of subjects from – at last count – 204 different nations and territories. When a group of scientists pulled together the project's most recent complete figures on infertility, covering a mere 198 countries, from 1990 to 2017, it found that over this period, infertility rates had increased for women by 0.37 per cent per year, on average, and 0.29 per cent a year for men.[1]

What did this mean? Infertility in this instance is defined as a failure to begin a pregnancy after a year of regular and unprotected sex. And to consider one of the increases, while 0.37 per cent might not sound much, the numbers add up, both over time and across a population. It means that, on average, the number of infertile women per 100,000 people rose by about 200 during the whole study period. Even using a fairly conservative estimate of the number of women of fertile age in the UK, that would be nearly 25,000 more women affected by infertility in one country alone.

Other research suggests that among couples actually trying to reproduce, somewhere between 8 per cent and 12 per cent experience problems. It is sometimes portrayed as an issue mainly in wealthier Western nations, but this is increasingly not the case. The Global Burden of Disease study found that the fastest increases in infertility were in Latin America, North Africa and the Middle East, and South-East Asia.[2] But again, if you are trying desperately to conceive, knowing other people face the same plight is not really a help. As the former British prime minister Harold Wilson once said about another predicament: if you don't have a job then it doesn't matter what the national unemployment statistics say – your own rate is 100 per cent.

Such was the case for Deborah. She and her partner had been trying to have a child for three years, without success. They were now considering going to a specialist fertility clinic or seeking IVF treatment, but she wanted to see first if stress could potentially be part of the picture. She arrived at the clinic feeling despondent and, as she put it, increasingly isolated.

The clinic is not a fertility clinic, although it has links with fertility specialists. But stress and wider metabolic health can play a big part in fertility, something Deborah knew only too well – she was, after all, a scientist. As a senior university lecturer in physics, cortisol was not her specialist subject, but she was very used to reading academic studies and had been doing a lot of her own research.

While the physiology and endocrinology behind female infertility is enormously complex, the wider risk-factors behind these are relatively well known. One is weight. Having a BMI of 30 or above has been shown to affect fertility, as can smoking and drinking too much alcohol. On these points, Deborah knew she was in the clear. A non-smoker who rarely drank, she was a healthy weight and still very fit, having regularly taken part in triathlons. Particularly high amounts of intensive exercise can affect ovulation and thus fertility, but Deborah knew this and had cut back her training regime when she and her partner started trying to conceive. She was now just fit, not superhumanly fit.

There were two other things to consider, one which she very obviously had no control over. Deborah was, at the time, thirty-six years old, and women's fertility tends to decline from their mid-thirties. One Chinese study into rising global infertility rates noted that one potential factor was likely to be the later age at which people decide to have children, a product of both social changes and, in countries like the UK, expensive housing making it harder for younger people to live together.

This could partly explain Deborah's situation. However, she first started trying to become pregnant at thirty-three, which by modern standards is not especially late – the average age of a British first-time mother is around thirty-one.

There was also stress, something Deborah knew more about than the average person arriving through the clinic doors. A voracious reader of books about psychotherapy, she knew her childhood was likely to have left her potentially more susceptible to its effects. Her parents had been, in her words, 'charming but utterly useless' – a mother who was a functioning alcoholic; a father who was not but was nonetheless completely unsuited to filling the void of domestic practicality and affection, let alone challenging his wife about her drinking. Deborah's younger brother had struggled with his mental health and drifted from job to job. She had always excelled at academia and sport, as much through sheer hard work as natural aptitude, a character trait she was keenly aware was likely to be as much of a coping mechanism as was her brother's flakiness.

Deborah was equally up to speed on the likely physiological implications of long-term stress and how these might affect fertility, coming to the clinic with a very clear plan for what she wanted, down to the specific tests. Her blood glucose was, as you might expect for someone so healthy, entirely normal. But her cortisol concentrations were elevated. She even opted to have a hair sample tested to gauge the measure over several months. Once again her hunch was right: her levels were above the norm.

This left an even greater conundrum than usually presented at the clinic. Deborah had a seemingly good idea about what the issue was, but what could she do next? Her extensive personal research meant she had already cut back on things she realized could increase her cortisol levels, particularly high-intensity exercise. She had also spent two years in psychotherapy, trying to better understand a background she had already thought about very deeply. What next? Ahead, there now seemed to be only an impasse.

Exactly how does stress affect fertility? In some ways this is fairly simple to explain, and in some broad ways familiar from earlier chapters. The hormones released by chronic stress, notably cortisol, have a tendency to make the homeostatic balance of the body work less well. And when it comes to conception, this balance is particularly delicate – and not just for women.

With female fertility, most people know about the two big hormonal players, oestrogen and progesterone. But there is also follicle-stimulating hormone, or FSH, which helps control the menstrual cycle; anti-mullerian hormone (AMH), which sustains eggs, the levels of which can be tested as a proxy for the number of eggs remaining; plus luteinizing hormone, or LH, which among other functions triggers ovulation. And there is something called gonadotropin-releasing hormone, which in yet another endocrine acronym is usually shortened to GnRH. This prompts the pituitary gland to produce and secrete LH and FSH. There is also a role for testosterone, which is not just involved in male sexual function.

Hormones

Oestrogen: A primary female sex hormone, this plays a central role in ovulation and the menstrual cycle, as well as puberty pregnancy and other elements of bodily function such as bone strength.

> **Progesterone:** This is also crucial to the menstrual cycle and to pregnancy. In the latter, it thickens the lining of the uterus, allowing an embryo to grow.
>
> **Testosterone:** The key sex hormone for men, it is involved in everything from sperm production to muscle mass. It also exists in women, albeit in lower concentrations, and is connected to sexual development and behaviour, as well as stronger bones.

Many female fertility problems are associated with insulin resistance, the common knock-on effect from chronically elevated cortisol. Overly high levels of insulin, produced to compensate for it working inefficiently, can cause women to release more testosterone, upsetting its balance with oestrogen. This can interfere with the work of LH on what are called granulosa cells, which are within the follicles, the tiny sacs that each contain an egg. This is the central element of the ovulation process, so high insulin can very much impede pregnancy.

New research has also linked insulin resistance to one of the more common medical causes of infertility, a condition called polycystic ovary syndrome, or PCOS, in which eggs are not properly released.[3] This affects about 1 in 10 women, and can often be treated with medication. New studies indicate that as many as 80 per cent of PCOS cases could be connected to insulin resistance.

PCOS is often associated with weight, as is insulin resistance, and weight can be one of the major barriers to fertility. But this was not the case for Deborah. She was not overweight, and remained sufficiently fit that it seemed less likely that insulin resistance was behind her inability thus far to conceive. But excess cortisol on its own can be enough. It can affect the way GnRH is released in pulses by the hypothalamus, the hormone control-box of the brain, which can then limit GnRH's effectiveness in the secretion of LH, which triggers ovulation. We know this in part because of various experiments on animals artificially doused with cortisol, and also because Cushing's syndrome, in which the body creates too much cortisol naturally, has been shown to impede the work of GnRH and therefore conception.

All this can seem quite technical, not to mention awash in confusing acronyms. Adding to the complications, researchers concede that they still don't fully understand quite how these effects play out. But the fact they happen appears in little doubt. So-called meta-studies, where researchers pull together years of research by others on a single subject to try to sum up the collective knowledge, have shown that in real-world studies, infertility in both men and women has tended to be associated with higher measured cortisol levels. This is, however, not an inevitability. What causal effect does exist seems to depend significantly on other factors, including genetics, people's overall health, and the way their body responds more generally to stress.

Another factor appears particularly significant for infertility and stress: how long the stress has lasted. It is chronic stress which apparently makes the difference. One British study which followed the fortunes of 135 women at an infertility clinic over nearly two years found that saliva tests for cortisol did not seem to correlate with the likelihood or not of getting pregnant, whether measured as waking cortisol or its trajectory over the whole day. However, with cortisol tests from hair samples, which can indicate levels experienced over several months, it was a different story. Women with elevated hair cortisol were between a quarter and a third less likely to become pregnant over the research period than those who did not.[4]

*

Deborah, ever the well-prepared overachiever, not only knew about much of this research, but arrived armed with a very good question, one to which there was no straightforward answer: how do you take into account the fact that infertility is, itself, a very stressful experience? Could that stress be part of the problem?

She recounted her own experiences: a decision to try for a baby which began as a hugely exciting joint adventure, but then became alternately a puzzle and almost a chore, and eventually a source of some tension and disagreement between Deborah and her partner. The build-up to her arrival at the clinic had been particularly fraught. Infertility is very much not a female-only affair. Depending on which study you read, the man can be solely the cause in anything from about 20 per cent to 40 per cent of infertility cases, and the issues can also often be joint. But – a narrative many infertility experts will be familiar with – Deborah's partner appeared convinced she was the problem, and had strongly encouraged her to pursue any possible answers, such as her own stress.

In yet another example of the cascading effects of stress, their arguments, Deborah said, had caused both of them to sleep less well than normal in recent months. This has been linked to yet more potential problems with infertility, for both women and men. Some studies have indicated that poor sleep could affect the quality of sperm, a major factor in male fertility issues. For women, research has shown that both less sleep and interrupted sleep patterns can trigger the HPA axis, increasing the amount of cortisol sloshing around the body, and separately can affect the delicate balance of hormones like LH and FSH. Yet another substance, thyroid-stimulating hormone, has been shown to rise significantly with lack of sleep, which can interfere with ovulation and disrupt menstruation more widely.

Deborah presented all this clearly and calmly. Both her scientific background and the way her personality had emerged from the chaos of her childhood made her very rational, approaching everything as a problem to be solved, a trait she understood was likely also to be a way to mask stress – a means to focus more on facts than emotions.

*

And this is yet another factor to take into account. As with everything else to do with stress, the way it affects fertility is not just about the sheer amount experienced, or for how long. You must also consider the person concerned.

While it would be foolish to view a particular personality type as more or less likely to become pregnant, there is a lot of research about the way predispositions to being affected by stress, often laid down in early childhood, play a big role in the physiological repercussions for fertility.

One example of this was a Swedish study which followed the fortunes of a group of women beginning IVF treatment. This in part sought to measure their stress through levels of cortisol and of prolactin, the latter being a hormone connected to lactation and breast development, where high levels can also be seen as a sign of stress. Another part of the research saw participants fill in questionnaires for a standard academic assessment of personality, and to indicate their levels of anxiety. It found that when measured against the results for a group of women who had been able to conceive, those starting IVF showed significantly greater levels of both cortisol and prolactin. It also concluded that while anxiety did not seem to be associated with infertility, this was very much the case for a wider tendency towards suspicion and guilt.[5] Such feelings, the researchers noted, could indicate that certain personality traits can have an impact on fertility – but equally, they could just be a product of the sheer strain of trying to have a child using IVF.

One of the problems with this sort of research is that infertility is often hidden, unless people seek help. For example, talking about it at the clinic had been the first time Deborah had discussed the three-year process with anyone except her partner. And, to be blunt, there are only so many IVF clinics at which you can find research subjects that you know for certain are facing fertility issues. Plus, sample sizes for these tend to be smaller and to be particular types of people.

Some broader studies have been attempted, with fascinating results. A Finnish project tracked a large group of women who had said they hoped to start a family, and then saw over time who did. Among the factors that made a successful pregnancy more likely, some were perhaps unsurprising, for example less tendency towards psychosomatic illness symptoms, a lack of recent negative life events, a stable body weight and not drinking too much coffee.[6] The advice for women seeking to become pregnant is to limit their caffeine intake, as too much can affect ovulation and increase the risks of miscarriage. Deborah, inevitably, knew all about this and had completely stopped drinking coffee. Other advantageous factors were a bit more unlikely-sounding, including being a youngest sibling and looking younger than your actual age.

This is all slightly muddy stuff, and was not a huge amount of help to Deborah. Her psychotherapy was intended to help her with stress, but she was aware she also had a tendency to sometimes not immediately trust people. She would sometimes feel guilty over matters about which she had limited or no control, such as her brother's latest mishaps. But this was long-term stuff, rooted in childhood. She worried that tackling it slowly via therapy could run up against the gradual but inexorable biological time constraints of trying to conceive.

Deborah was, however, unapologetic about one emotion: she was deeply annoyed with her partner for refusing to engage with the idea he might be behind the fertility problem, whether wholly or in part.

Men and fertility

While the male contribution to pregnancy is in some ways more biologically straightforward, not to mention short-lived, it is just as reliant on homeostasis and thus equally as susceptible to the destabilizing effects of lifestyle and stress. The standard gauge of male fertility is sperm concentration and the regularity of sperm shape. The means by which stress can seemingly undermine this are many and not completely understood.

One of the less complex interactions is the way that cortisol and other glucocorticoids can affect the production of testosterone in what are known as Leydig cells, within the testes, which secrete and synthesize sex hormones called androgens, the main one being testosterone.

Another possible factor appears to be the impact of stress hormones on something called nectin-3, which sounds like a minor planet from *Star Wars* but is in fact a protein which has a major role in the development of sperm. Studies have shown that particularly chronic stress can impair its function, with a potential knock-on effect for sperm effectiveness. Other studies indicate that stress can hamper the function of Sertoli cells, which are within the testes and play a vital role in sperm formation.

Once again, away from the mechanics of *how* this might happen, the fact that it *does* happen has been shown clearly and repeatedly. Since measuring sperm quality is simpler than assessing the various elements of female fertility, it can be more easily monitored as the result of a particular external stress, separate from the specifics of couples trying to conceive. One refreshingly simple study took a group of Dutch male medical students and tested their sperm at the start of the academic year, then shortly before their annual exams and again during the middle of the exam period. They were all instructed to abstain from any sexual activity for at least 48 hours beforehand, something which would have been a challenge of varying difficulties for a collection of young men. The findings were clear: both just before and during the exams, sperm concentration was notably decreased compared to the non-stressed period, as was the straightness of the sperm.[7]

There is an entire sub-genre of fertility studies which looks at the impact on sperm of that most dramatically stressful of situations: war. War is such a distilled invocation of stress that it can sometimes feel that the moment a conflict breaks out, just behind the tanks and the aid workers come groups of university academics, rounding up civilians to examine everything from the psychological impacts to cortisol concentrations and, in a few cases, sperm quality. More often, for understandable reasons, the research takes place retrospectively. One relatively recent study used a cache of stored semen samples dating back decades at the American University of Beirut Medical Center to examine the impact of the chaotic and often very brutal Lebanese Civil War of 1975–1990, in which an estimated 150,000 people died. This compared more than 4,500 samples given during 1985–1989, with 6,200 given during 1991–1995, when peace had returned. On average, the wartime sperm concentrations were significantly lower.[8]

It is an effect which can linger. One US project used sperm samples from several hundred veterans of the Vietnam war and compared them with those of similar men who had not served. Even many years after the conflict was over, the veterans' sperm concentrations were, on average, considerably lower.[9]

It does appear that for stress to have this sort of impact it needs to be either sustained or highly acute, or both. One long-term study of a group of men found minimal evidence of everyday work stress affecting sperm quality, whereas the recent death of a close family member did have an impact.[10]

Stress and your baby's gender

One of the more curious-seeming impacts of particularly severe stress, such as that caused by wars and natural disasters, is that it can skew the overall birth rate towards more girls being born, against fewer boys. This has been shown by researchers a number of times.

One particularly well-known study found a notable drop-off in male births in the wake of the devastating earthquake in 1995 in Kobe, Japan, in which around 6,000 people died and tens of thousands were made homeless.[11] Later research found the same effect in the wake of the September 11 attacks on New York City,[12] and even, to a lesser extent, in the UK after the Covid pandemic.[13]

The reason for this appears to be that extreme stress can make it more likely that if a woman has a miscarriage in the early stages

> of pregnancy, this will affect a male foetus rather than a female one. This seems to be an automatic bodily response based on the fact that male foetuses are less resilient but also grow larger, requiring more bodily resources from the mother, which the body believes could be difficult in a crisis.
>
> Unlike the impact of stress on fertility, this gender split seems to be a product of brief, intense worry rather than something long-standing. One study even found a change in the gender ratio in the very specific cohort of Slovenian children conceived around the time of the country's extremely short war of independence from the then-crumbling Yugoslav state, in the summer of 1991.
>
> Lasting just ten days in June and July, this was a proper war, with around eighty people killed, but it ended rapidly, with Yugoslav forces surrendering, after which Slovenia was allowed to declare its independence. And yet, in the six to nine months after the conflict, the ratio of boys to girls was lower than would be expected.[14]

When it came to the puzzle of Deborah's inability thus far to conceive, any information about the male side of the equation was, inevitably, only known second-hand. But Deborah was treating the situation as if it was a physics equation to be unlocked, and was happy to present all the facts she had. Her partner had not suffered a bereavement – nor, indeed, had he been involved in a war – and while he could have a tendency to be stubborn and closed-off, as shown by his insistence that the fertility issue was hers to resolve, she believed he suffered less obviously from stress than her. His parents had been loving and stable, even if the default family approach was somewhere between uncomplaining and repressed.

She did, however, have one possible clue: while she had cut back on her exercise regime to try to boost their chances of conceiving, her partner was coping with the strain of their long wait by doing more and more. He was, when she first came to the clinic, training for an ultra-endurance triathlon called an Ironman, where a

2.4-mile open-water swim is followed by a 112-mile bike ride and then, to cap things off, a full marathon. People do extremely well to complete an Ironman in twelve hours. It often takes them much longer.

Many studies have shown that very intense exercise can have an effect on menstruation and thus women's fertility, even if a fair bit of this effect seems to be also predicated on body weight and the age at which the sport was taken up. One showed that, among fourteen-year-old girls, while 95 per cent of a control group had gone through puberty, for high-level runners the equivalent figure was 40 per cent, and for gymnasts it was just 20 per cent.[15]

For men, the correlation appears less fixed, although some studies have shown that particularly strenuous and long-lasting exercise can seemingly have an effect on sperm quality. Perhaps more importantly for Deborah, whose partner was going out for long training rides every weekend, very extended sports cycling is also linked to male infertility, potentially as a result of sustained scrotal heat, which is also not especially good for sperm.

There are no simple answers

In several ways, Deborah was an unusual client. People generally arrive at the clinic, irrespective of the issue which brought them there, seeking medical answers. Deborah not only knew the science almost as well as the clinic team, she came in the expectation of something slightly different: confirmation that there wasn't necessarily an answer.

Deborah realized that while she had made many efforts to both limit the amount of stress she faced and mitigate its impact on her body, she was most likely the sort of person with a particular susceptibility to cortisol. She also knew that this was something not easily undone. But before she and her partner decided on whether they wanted to go down the never-straightforward route of specialist medical fertility help and then, potentially, IVF, she first wanted to know whether her cortisol was elevated, and if so, whether there was anything she had missed to improve her fertility – if, indeed, she was the issue.

Deborah said that, for now, she would not take up the offer to be put in touch with a dedicated fertility expert. She and her partner were going to have a think. And that, it seemed, was it. Until eighteen months later.

The news came in an email, one that began, in a typically understated way, with Deborah's apology for passing on news that might not be of interest. Quite the opposite. She was pregnant, and not through IVF or any kind of treatment.

Deeply bruised by the previous three years, and worried for their relationship, she and her partner had – and these were her words – 'decided to give up'. They took the conscious decision to think and act as if they would never become parents and try to look at the positives. They took long holidays using money Deborah had set aside in case she did not meet the criteria for NHS IVF treatment or if she wanted to undergo more than the three cycles offered. She started drinking coffee again. Her partner completed the Ironman and took a break from exercise to – again in her words – 'eat more good food'. And then one day, without having previously even noted the timing, she realized her period was already over a week late.

People often tend to couch such unexpected pregnancies as near-miracles, something with no rational explanation. And the truth is that even the most experienced fertility expert can often be utterly flummoxed by such end stories, both positive and negative. But in this case, there were definitely a few pointers from science.

The most obvious was the idea that Deborah's stress and subsequent cortisol levels might not have been entirely the product of her difficult childhood: the sheer strain of trying to get pregnant, and the impact it had on her relationship, could well have played a part. Her partner dialling-down his very intense exercise might also have helped – the studies show that, particularly with men and their sperm quality, when such exertion does have an impact, this effect tends to wear off fairly quickly.

But there could also have been something else in the mix, about which Deborah was silent in her email – it would very much not be her style to mention it – but which can play a big role in such sudden pregnancies. It sounds almost too obvious to be true, but they might just have been having more sex.

It is too simplistic to say that people automatically have less sex when they are stressed. The studies are mixed, and some involving young women have shown that those with signs of stress, even depression, sometimes have sex more often, on average, than their peers who do not.[16] That said, a slightly clinical-sounding experiment in which a group of women were shown a pornographic film while having physiological signs of sexual arousal measured found that those who tested for higher levels of cortisol were less stimulated.[17]

But sex as a procreational chore, especially if repeated over a long period, can diminish the charm. Sometimes it is better when the pressure is off. And just maybe that was the case for Deborah.

Procreation is, of course, even more complex and varied than a single chapter with one case study can properly set out. We have seen the many ways stress can impact male and female fertility through the example of a heterosexual couple having unprotected sex. There are, very obviously, many other types of couple and family, and other ways people try to conceive, not least IVF and the use of donated sperm or eggs. The endocrinology remains broadly the same, but – as mentioned repeatedly in this book – the way it manifests is never the same twice.

So far we have alluded several times to one of the primary reasons why the same hormones can affect people in such wildly different ways: the impact of their upbringing, particularly in infancy and early childhood. This can be a difficult subject to consider. But it is utterly central to our story.

CHAPTER 9

Love, Touch and Inheritance: Early Years and Stress

This is a chapter about long-term consequences: how our very earliest years, including in the womb, can have an impact for the rest of our lives. Much of this is often felt through physical health, and within this, stress and its manifestations are often of particular importance.

As such, this is a chapter which could, for some readers, provoke intense feelings. Some parts might feel painfully relevant to your direct experiences, whether as child, a parent or carer, or in another role.

So before we dive into the research, let us remind ourselves of the most important message of all from this book. This is not about guilt. There are, as we are about to see, much bigger forces at work. Highlighting research which shows that some events can have long-term consequences should never be a matter for shame. This is simply about understanding.

And in another repeated motif of this book, these bigger forces are often both various and almost inevitably beyond any individual's control. All this is something Joeli Brearley knows only too well.

When Brearley first knew she was having a child, she was happily working with a children's charity and had secured funding for a project that would give her an income throughout her pregnancy. She let the charity know her news, assuring them she would be perfectly able to complete the scheme as planned. But then events took an unexpected turn.

'The next day they left a voicemail saying, "We're going to pull your contract, please hand everything over immediately,"' she says. 'It was very obvious why they were doing it. And that left me in a really difficult situation – I didn't have an income and I was four months pregnant.'

There are laws across the world to protect someone from being discriminated against on the grounds of pregnancy, and Brearley was confident the decision contravened these. She found a lawyer and considered taking the charity to an industrial tribunal, which hear claims of unfair dismissal, but was alarmed to learn their fee to represent her would be around £9,000.

As she considered her next move, a routine hospital check-up uncovered a problem with her cervix, making the pregnancy very high-risk, with a chance her baby could be born prematurely – something she was told was very likely connected to stress. Brearley underwent an operation and was sent home with some very stern advice: 'The doctor told me, "The main thing you need to do is don't get stressed. It's stress that has probably caused this. It's stress that will make it worse. Do everything you can to avoid stress." And I was like, "Yeah, right."'

Brearley spent the next three weeks she recounts 'lying on the sofa, either crying or rubbing my belly, and begging my unborn child not to come out anytime soon. I'd lost my job, I'd lost my income and I'd lost any semblance of a career. I was having to rely on my parents.'

In the end, the pregnancy progressed well and Brearley is now mother to, as she puts it, 'a very healthy ten-year-old boy'. By the time she gave birth, the three-month limit to begin tribunal proceedings had lapsed, so she dropped the idea of taking action against the charity. But this was not the end. Speaking to other mothers at parent-and-baby groups, Brearley said she was 'absolutely astounded by how many said to me that they had really bad experiences at work from the point that they said they were pregnant – harassment, bullying, lack of promotion opportunities, being sidelined.' And so she set up a website dedicated to collating such stories. This is now a campaigning charity with the very memorable name of Pregnant Then Screwed.

Brearley's story offers several lessons. One is that stress can affect women in very particular ways, partly because of biology but also due to societal inequalities. This is, very obviously, one part of a wider issue. As we saw earlier, there are reams of studies setting out the ways that people from minority ethnic backgrounds can experience above-average levels of stress, with the same true for people with disabilities. But when it comes to women and pregnancy, there is also very strong evidence that severe stress at this time can have a notable effect on the unborn child, both in terms of how the infant physically develops and their lifelong susceptibility to stress, and thus ailments connected to stress. This does not end with birth. The early years of childhood can also be utterly pivotal for something as physiologically basic as how much cortisol someone secretes as an adult, and how much it then affects them.

There is another very important point to note, one also illustrated by Brearley's story. This is not direct causation, an inevitable cascade of events. It is simply about vulnerability factors. Statistically, a child exposed to foetal and infant stress will be more likely to be affected in adulthood. But that is a matter of averages, not destiny, and many other things are involved. Brearley's son, she says, appears to have been unscathed by what she went through.

Another vital piece of context is that while this narrative is primarily considered in the context of mothers, there is very clearly more to it. Plenty of research shows that fathers, and other family members or caregivers, can have hugely significant impact, whether positive or negative. But whatever the cause, the consequences can be very, very real.

The lost ledgers

One of the most pivotal breakthroughs in understanding how infancy can shape future life abruptly announced itself when an eminent British epidemiologist pulled his car into the driveway of his rural home in Hampshire at some speed and amid much excitement. David Barker rushed into the house and told his wife, Jan, to leave their several children for a few minutes and get into the car with him, as he had something to show her. He parked in a nearby farm gateway and pulled out a small red book with a very battered cover. This was the evidence he had spent years looking for, and it changed our understanding of long-term health for ever.

The unprepossessing volume was an official record of infant deaths and their locations in England and Wales near the start of the twentieth century. Barker, who had spent years studying health inequalities, was examining it in his office when he realized that most of the areas it listed as having particularly high infant mortality rates still did when he was reading it several decades on, in the early 1980s. There was a pattern – but what was it?

This was the genesis of something now known as the Barker Theory of Foetal Programming, the idea that adverse circumstances when a baby is in the womb can have an impact which lasts for life. His idea was based around physical health, notably connected to poor maternal nutrition, but it laid the groundwork for decades of subsequent research which showed that mental stresses can have a similar effect.

A few years later, in the mid-1980s, Barker uncovered an even more remarkable set of books, which provided part of the answer to this mysterious pattern. These were long-forgotten ledgers recording almost all births in the English county of Hertfordshire from 1911 to 1938, listing for each baby a series of personal details plus their weight when they were born and their weight aged one. This was, it turned out, the work of the slightly formidable Ethel Burnside, Hertfordshire's first chief health visitor, who assembled a team of midwives to make home visits, each one armed with a set of spring-weighted scales. Burnside played her part too, in one year totalling nearly 3,000 miles of travel between appointments on her bike.

This was a goldmine of information, and not just about regional trends but identifiable individuals. Barker and his team set about tracing the men from that cohort – tracing women from an era in which the majority married and changed their surnames was more difficult – if they were still living, or their death records if they were not, which they managed to do in 5,654 cases. The findings were remarkable. Of the 1,186 men who had died, 434 had done so due to heart disease. And the correlation with weight in infancy was very clear: the men who, as one-year-olds, had weighed 8kg or less were almost three times more likely to have died from heart disease than those who had weighed 12kg or more.[1] Subsequent analysis of those still alive showed that both low birth weights and low weight at one year also gave a much greater likelihood of the men having high blood pressure or type 2 diabetes. As the headline of an article Barker wrote for the *British Medical Journal* put it, 'The womb may be more important than the home.'

*

This has relevance to the study of stress for two reasons. The first is that stress has been shown to be a factor behind low birth weights, whether at full term or because the baby was born prematurely. The most thorough examination of this effect, a meta-study which compiled data from thirty-one projects covering a total of more than 5.5 million women, found that very stressful events when a woman was pregnant gave a 23 per cent higher chance of a low birth weight – defined as less than 2.5 kg (about 5.5lb) – and a 20 per cent chance that the baby was born before thirty-seven weeks.[2]

Barker's insights also provided a scientific basis for ideas which had already emerged from psychotherapy, which argued that much about the way an adult turned out, including how they coped with stress, was fashioned in the early years of life, not least in the womb.

We saw in Chapter 8 how persistently high concentrations of cortisol in the blood can make it more difficult to conceive a child; it can then also make it harder for the embryo to develop. Tests on rats have shown that artificially administered cortisol seems to block the way oestrogen helps the growth of the uterus, vital for healthy offspring. Other studies have demonstrated that high levels of artificial glucocorticoids can impede the progress of mice embryos.

It is about more than just birth weight, even if that can sometimes be a useful shorthand for the cumulative ill effects. Years of studies have shown that significant maternal stress can cause what is termed developmental programming, in which the baby develops differently in the womb, making them more at risk in adulthood from ailments including type 2 diabetes, high blood pressure, emotional and cognitive issues, and obesity. Much of this, it seems, is due to the infant's HPA axis being set to a higher sensitivity, the result of greater exposure to cortisol, notably in parts of the developing body rich in glucocorticoid receptors, such as the liver, brain and fat tissue. There is increasing evidence that a lot of this process is epigenetic – that is, causing modifications to the baby's DNA.

Yet again, it is about the extent and duration of exposure. Glucocorticoids play a vital role in helping infants in the womb prepare for birth, maturing their tissues and organs, especially the lungs. This is why artificial cortisol-related steroids are given to women at risk of premature birth. The problem is when the infant's system becomes overloaded.

Malnutrition during pregnancy seems to create a particularly high foetal exposure to cortisol. A whole series of studies have been based around Dutch people born between the winter of 1944 and the spring of 1945, when the delayed liberation by Allied forces in the Second World War saw a famine take hold of what has otherwise been a largely well-fed country, with official rations in some places falling to between 400 and 800 calories a day. The impact on the children depended in part on when their mothers lacked food. Babies exposed to malnutrition later during the pregnancy tended to be born smaller, and as adults showed a greater propensity towards glucose intolerance and type 2 diabetes. Those who experienced it in early gestation were more likely to be a normal weight, but the repercussions after they grew up seemed even greater: as well as showing a heightened risk of obesity, they had three times the incidence of heart disease than non-famine children.

The reasons for all this are varied. As well as increased maternal cortisol, the insulin-connected part of the pancreas appears to develop particularly late in gestation, which could explain the impaired glucose tolerance of those whose mothers were hungry during that period. Scientists also found epigenetic changes related to metabolism and growth. You can see why this would have a lifelong impact.

David Barker also noted the impact of nutrition in his work, attributing some of the differences in health outcomes he found between various English towns and cities to the differing qualities of diets available to pregnant women decades earlier. He subsequently worked in the US and studied the so-called Stroke Belt in a cluster of southern states, where there is an unusually high level of strokes and other cardiovascular ailments, beyond what would be expected, given the states' demographics and living standards. This, Barker believed, was the long-term legacy of malnutrition following the US Civil War a century before.

Why was London so healthy?

One of the many puzzles looked at by David Barker in his examination of differing death rates across English regions was the anomaly of London. At the time he was researching the subject, in the 1980s, people living in big UK cities tended to have above-average mortality rates – apart from in London. In none of London's boroughs, he found, were cardiovascular death rates above the national average.

Barker's ingenious theory was that this was a product of the Victorian era, when many London mothers were healthy, young, rural women who had arrived in the capital to work as servants. They had been brought up outside the city's squalor, and as servants they

> tended to be better fed than most other working-class Londoners. And so they went on to have healthy children, who were now growing old in better-than-average health. This idea was backed up by health statistics from the era, Barker discovered. In the early years of the twentieth century, the city's rates of maternal mortality and death in early infancy were also well below the national average.
>
> Barker quoted Charles Booth, the Victorian social reformer who plotted poverty maps of London, in describing how this never-ending stream of sturdy rural recruits seemingly kept the city going: 'London is to a great extent nourished by the literal consumption of bone and sinew from the country; by the absorption every year of large numbers of persons of stronger physique . . . only to give place in their turn to a fresh set of recruits, after London life for one or two generations has reduced them to the level of those among whom they live.'[3]

The importance of touch

In 1956 a US psycho-biologist called Seymour Levine, whose work helped advance many of Hans Selye's ideas about stress, discovered something in an experiment which seemed fairly unusual. He and his co-researchers took litters of very young rat pups, who had not yet been weaned, and put them through one of three sets of experiences. A first group was taken from their mothers for a few minutes every day and placed in a special chamber to be given mild electric shocks, before being returned. Another group was also moved away from their mothers briefly but not given shocks. The third was not handled at all. This daily regime lasted for three weeks. Two months later, the now adult animals – growing up is a swift business in the rat world – were put through a series of cognitive and behavioural tests, including how long it took them to find their way out of the unlocked door of a cage to escape a loud buzzer noise, and the way they behaved when the way out was blocked.

The team found that both in terms of speed of learning and behaviour, the latter measured by how often they froze in fright, the rats who were handled and shocked, and the rats who were just handled, performed notably better than the ones who were never touched.[4] It might seem that being picked up by a giant hand and removed from your mother when you are a tiny rat pup would seem more frightening than soothing, but Levine explained this as being the result of the extra licking and grooming that the pups received from their mothers when they were returned.

Subsequent studies have examined footage of rat pups with their mothers and found that those paid the most attention seem to be more relaxed when placed in a stressful situation – and, crucially, secrete about half as much cortisol and other stress hormones.[5] Early parental focus seems crucial, to the extent of even compensating for a regime of electric shocks.

Two years later, another American academic, the psychologist Harry Harlow, showed just how vital this bond of touch was for infants in a study which these days would presumably never make it past the first meeting of the university ethics board. He removed baby rhesus monkeys from their mothers a few hours after they were born and put them in a cage with two substitute 'mothers', both crudely-made inanimate models. One had a body of exposed wire, but with a baby bottle of milk attached to it. The other provided no nourishment but the wire body was covered in a soft, fleecy cloth. In every case, the infant monkey would feed from the wire-bodied only 'mother' but spent much more time with the cloth-covered version. Photos show the tiny, wide-eyed monkeys clinging to the cloth body, which is topped with a sinister-looking robotic head, one clearly fashioned from spare parts lying around the laboratory. The pictures are easily searchable online, but this is not necessarily recommended unless you want to feel heartbroken on the infant monkeys' behalf.

In another test, Harlow and his team placed the monkeys in a strange room, sometimes with their cloth 'mother' and sometimes alone. In the first situation, they would use it as a base from which to explore the room, returning regularly for comfort. But without the surrogate mother they would be visibly distressed, rocking and crying.[6]

*

Appallingly, there are real-life human examples of what happens when babies and infants are deprived of touch and nurture. Perhaps the most eloquent if depressing are studies of children kept in the vast state-run orphanages of Romania during the long rule of the communist dictator Nicolae Ceaușescu. After he was overthrown in 1989, charity workers found rooms of infants and babies who were fed and bathed according to a rigid schedule but otherwise left entirely alone. Studies of the children as they grew up found a range of behavioural and even cerebral issues, but most notably a disrupted supply of cortisol. A loving adoptive family could address many of the problems, with the best results coming from an early removal from neglect, but cortisol remained in flux. One of the many complexities of this process is that while a lesser degree of dysfunction in infancy tends to bring a tendency towards elevated cortisol, in cases as bad as this it can at times instead flatten supply of the hormone, a factor often linked to later depression. However, the lesson is fundamentally the same: in infancy, we very obviously require sustenance – but comfort and touch are almost equally vital for development.

Unpicking the health consequences of all this can be difficult, in part because unpleasant young-life events can also make people more susceptible to choices which can harm them. A US study of nearly 10,000 people found that when they were asked about a series of childhood experiences ranging from abuse to living with domestic violence or addiction, there was a clear correlation between reporting more than one of these and experiencing ill health as an adult – but also more likelihood that the person ended up smoking, using drugs or drinking to excess, or being physically inactive or obese.[7] Once again, it can be a vicious cycle.

The Adverse Childhood Experiences Study

One of the most vivid illustrations of how much our childhoods shape our future health was a study conducted over twenty-five years ago which is still sometimes used as a broad diagnostic tool.

The Adverse Childhood Experiences, or ACE, test asks people just ten questions about their life before the age of eighteen, covering experiences of psychological, physical, or sexual abuse, household violence, addiction or mental illness, imprisonment and divorce. Having been devised by a group of US researchers, they first put the test to 9,500 adults, who were also then asked about their health.

The results were striking: compared with those who had not suffered any of the experiences, those who reported four or more of them were between four and twelve times more likely to experience alcoholism, drug abuse, depression and attempted suicide as adults, as well as having a greater chance of overall poor health and severe obesity. Subsequent research has found a particularly close link with obesity, even for people who have faced fewer than four such experiences.[8]

It's easy enough to find the ACE test online, with plenty of resources available to help you interpret your results. Bear in mind, however, that it is a fairly basic metric. It takes no account of either adverse factors outside the home, or potentially positive ones inside it. It is not a marker of inescapable destiny, just a statistical indicator.

The impact of childhood does not necessarily have to involve anything as extreme as abuse, or starting life in a Romanian orphanage. Numerous studies have shown that even much more everyday parental neglect or chaos in infancy can bring subsequent difficulties regulating cortisol and thus coping with stress. As we saw in Chapter 4, studies have shown an apparent correlation between the parental warmth young people receive when growing up and the levels of cortisol they produce when facing stress. We also heard about the societally contested idea that cortisol can be elevated in infants who attend nurseries.

This is a realm of research where endocrinology, neuroscience and psychology cross over with the slightly more scientifically indistinct disciplines of psychotherapy and psychoanalysis. And in many ways, psychoanalysis got there first.

Less sentimentality and more spanking

For what might seem a surprisingly long period in the twentieth century, the idea of parents being affectionate towards their children was not just uncommon, it was in many instances openly discouraged. In 1928 John B. Watson, a leading US psychologist of his era, wrote a guide to child-rearing which included this very firm advice: 'Never hug and kiss them, never let them sit in your lap. If you must, kiss them once on the forehead when they say goodnight. Shake hands with them in the morning. When you are tempted to pet your child remember that mother love is a dangerous instrument.'[9]

Watson was no outlier. Writing slightly earlier, Granville Stanley Hall, who pioneered child psychology in the US, was if anything even more blunt. 'All that rot they teach to children about the little raindrop fairies with their buckets washing down the window panes must go,' he advised. 'We need less sentimentality and more spanking.'[10] Yet another well-known expert of the time, paediatrician Luther Emmett Holt, produced his own guide to child-rearing which described crying as 'the baby's exercise', adding: 'Babies under six months old should never be played with, and the less of it at any time the better for the infant.'[11]

This was, it should be noted, advice mainly aimed at the middle classes and better-off, and many homes of the period did see much physical affection. But it was an atmosphere which would have been highly familiar to John Bowlby, the creator of an entirely opposite philosophy, one he called 'attachment theory'.

Born in 1907, Bowlby was the son of a senior military doctor, Anthony Bowlby, who spent a time as surgeon to the royal family and was often away for long periods; his mother Mary came from a minor aristocratic family. In common with the practice of many English upper-class families of the era, the young John and his five siblings would have been almost strangers to their parents. His mother would visit the nursery briefly after breakfast, and read to the children when they were brought downstairs for an hour at 5 p.m. Bowlby was sent to a boarding school aged seven.

All this might seem a recipe for a notably disturbed childhood, but in a prelude to the idea that a positive attachment figure does not necessarily have to be the mother, Bowlby and his siblings had a long-serving nanny, who would have represented some consistency. Either way, Bowlby emerged with a very obvious ability to think for himself. After initially studying medicine at university, he switched to psychology, then taught for a period in what was described as 'a school for maladjusted children', where he first encountered the notion that such troubled youngsters very often seemed to have endured a chaotic or otherwise difficult infancy. He decided to return to medical school and train first as a psychiatrist and then as a psychoanalyst.

The idea of someone's early years being pivotal to their life was, of course, nothing new in the psychoanalytic world. But Bowlby rejected Sigmund Freud's notion that babies attach to their mother because she meets their orally-fixated needs, along with other feelings based on nascent sexuality. Melanie Klein, another major figure in psychoanalysis, had introduced the idea of the very early period of life being vital, but again with a focus on the baby's relationship with the mother through the breast. Bowlby felt both versions lacked a scientific basis.

Building on his work at the reform school, Bowlby studied a group of young thieves aged between five and sixteen at a centre for what were known then as juvenile delinquents, learning that seventeen of the forty-four had experienced prolonged separation from their mothers before the age of five. Of those seventeen, he deemed fifteen to be 'affectionless psychopaths', meaning they felt no remorse for their crimes.

By 1940, Bowlby had become convinced about the basics of a theory he would spend the rest of his career developing, writing in a psychoanalytic journal: 'If it became a tradition that small children were never subjected to complete or prolonged separation from their parents, in the same way that regular sleep and orange juice have become nursery traditions, I believe that many cases of neurotic character development would be avoided.'[12]

He went on to become a well-known expert on child development, with his 1951 guide to the subject being translated into ten languages. A year later he helped change the outdated rules under which English hospitals routinely banned or severely limited parental access to paediatric wards, even for very tiny children, co-making a film called *A Two Year Old Goes to Hospital*. This showed, in unflinching detail, the very obvious distress of a girl called Laura who had to spend eight days on a ward for a minor operation and did not understand why her mother could not be there with her. As with the image of the rhesus monkey clinging to its cloth mother, the forty-five-minute film is easily findable online; once again, that is not necessarily a recommendation to do this. It is a difficult watch.[13]

Bowlby did not begin to formally set out his ideas as a unifying theory until he had turned fifty, doing so in a series of lectures and then academic papers. Openly acknowledging the influence of Harry Harlow's rhesus monkey experiments, he summarized it thus: 'All of us, from the cradle to the grave, are happiest when life is organized as a series of excursions, long or short, from the secure base provided by the attachment figure.'[14]

Arguing that the idea of instinctive attachment originated in protection from predators, and is demonstrated by the way female apes carry around their young, Bowlby's view was that babies learned their sense of self from the continuity of the attachment-giver's smell, then their face, and the way expressions like smiles were mirrored between the two. Those who had such a model were, as Bowlby put it, securely attached – going into the world with the 'internal working model' of a responsive, reliable, loving caregiver, which provided them with a self they saw as worthy of attention and love. This framework was then used for a lifetime of other trusting relationships. Where the structure failed, he said, people were insecurely attached in one of three ways: avoidant, ambivalent or disorganized.

These categories were tested by his colleague and co-researcher, the US-Canadian psychologist Mary Ainsworth, who devised something called the Strange Situation test in the late 1960s. This begins with an infant aged about one and their primary caregiver playing in an unfamiliar room. What follows is a series of carefully choreographed events, including a stranger who arrives and starts to join the play, the caregiver leaving for a brief period and returning, and at one point the child being left alone for a short time. A securely attached child, the theory goes, uses their caregiver as this secure base to explore the new environment, engaging interactively with both them and the stranger. They will show some distress when the caregiver leaves but are swiftly comforted when they return. Depending on the type of insecure attachment, less secure infants may show intense distress, or indifference to the caregiver when they return.[15]

Attachment theory is undoubtedly thoughtful and nuanced, not to mention a massive shift forward from earlier views about parent–child ties – not just the 'less sentimentality and more spanking' approach of the early twentieth century but also many of the ideas in vogue when Bowlby set out his idea in the late 1950s. It has also been backed up, at least in part, by subsequent studies. Researchers have carried out the Strange Situation test with the add-on of saliva cortisol tests for the infants. This found that securely attached children have a strong but short-lived cortisol burst when the caregiver leaves the room, while for the insecurely attached ones this increase in cortisol is sustained – potentially setting in train a lifetime of higher stress-hormone levels. There are, however, significant criticisms. One is that the studies cited to back up Bowlby's ideas tend to have small sample sizes, as well as results which are often arguably as much a product of interpretation as reasoning.

One of the main critics of Bowlby's ideas was Michael Rutter, the pioneer of child psychiatry in the UK, who argued that early separation from the caregiver did risk difficulties, but was not necessarily life-defining. Rutter later carried out a major study of the children in Romanian orphanages and concluded that while the damage was very real, the majority nonetheless made significant improvements when they were given nurture. Rutter said that, to his credit, Bowlby had listened to the new evidence and adapted his ideas. The first few months and years, Rutter insisted, were not necessarily an inescapable destiny.

There is, of course, another big issue, one particularly relevant for this chapter. In outlining attachment theory, we have used 'caregiver', the standard term used these days. But Bowlby did not. His attachment figure was almost always the mother. Is it really a mother's fault if a child grows up insecurely attached, or plagued by stress and attendant ill health? That can sometimes seem to be the message, and it is one heavily freighted with stigma and guilt. There is, however, a lot more to it.

Within just a few years of Bowlby setting out his ideas, this relentless focus on the mother was already being robustly challenged by Margaret Mead, a pioneering US cultural anthropologist who argued that lots of other cultures did things differently. In many places, she said, child-rearing was a fundamentally more collective enterprise. Bowlby, Mead added, was trying to 'pin women down in their own homes'.[16]

Other critics have made similar points. Another eminent anthropologist, Sarah Hrdy, took issue with Bowlby's notion that because apes have continuous skin-to-skin contact between mothers and their infants, this must have been the way early humans existed. In fact, Hrdy noted, not even apes routinely do it, with about half of ape species farming out care of the young to the shared group – much, she argued, like modern humans use nurseries or ask their extended family to help. There was, she said, no evidence that children could not securely attach to a series of figures.[17]

In fairness to Bowlby – Hrdy, as well as other critics, acknowledge this – he did not insist on the complete primacy of the mother and also argued for the professionalization of childcare. However, his ideas have undeniably sometimes been used to make arguments which could well leave many women feeling trapped, guilty, or both.

In the US in particular, much of this has centred around a debate dubbed the Daycare Wars, sparked by the research of Jay Belsky, a child psychologist. In the 1980s he used Mary Ainsworth's Strange Situation test to conclude that infants around a year old who had twenty or more hours of childcare a week were more likely to be insecurely attached. Critics complained that this did not take into account either the quality of the childcare or the family situation.

A later study led by Belsky, which tracked over 1,300 children and their families in ten different parts of the US from birth, provided a more nuanced picture. When the children were just over four, an initial report found, those who had been in good-quality childcare tended to have slightly better language skills and cognition, but also more behavioural problems. A follow-up study when the same children were fifteen found much the same thing. The effects, Belsky and his co-researchers argued, are relatively small but 'they should not be dismissed'.[18]

The 'good enough mother'

Another totemic figure in the liaison between the science of the early years and psychoanalysis was Donald Winnicott, a near-contemporary of Bowlby who exerted a strong influence on him. Winnicott's work contains a hugely important message for this chapter: parental perfection is not only impossible, it could even be damaging.

> Winnicott's highly evocative and in many ways reassuring central idea was of the 'good enough mother', one who is emotionally available to their infant, but not to the exclusion of all else. This was, he argued, particularly relevant beyond the initial stage of babyhood. It was, he believed, useful for infants to understand that not all their needs would be met immediately and without question. Some frustration, whether in wanting to be fed or to have a toy passed to them, is a thing infants must learn to tolerate, in limited quantities, particularly if they can be confident their needs will be met in the end.[19]
>
> This helps the infant gradually develop a sense of self, Winnicott believed, something which would not happen if every moment of distress or frustration was alleviated immediately. The idea, first out in 1953, and which clearly has lessons for caregivers beyond the mother, is in many ways a hugely powerful one. As any first-time parent soon learns, mistakes will be made. The idea that this is not only inevitable, but in some ways beneficial, can be both reassuring and sanity-maintaining.

Where do the childcare wars leave us in a modern world in which about three quarters of British mothers with dependent children have jobs, and where statutory maternity leave lasts less than a year, the bulk of it paying, at the time of writing, a maximum of £184.03 a week?[20] Will returning to work really leave your child with a lifetime of cortisol overload? One very obvious answer is that none of this is a zero-sum game. Yes, there is some evidence related to different outcomes from some forms of childcare. But it will also not do your child's HPA axis much good to have as their attachment figure a mother who bitterly resents not being able to work, or where both parents are hugely stressed as they cannot pay the bills. Plus, there is another thing to take into account, one largely absent from the early papers on attachment theory: fathers.

Bowlby himself had four children, but in an echo of his own

childhood he was not a natural parent and played a very limited role in their upbringing. Seventy or so years on, things are different in many ways, if not all. For example, in the UK fathers can now play a more central role in the first year of their child's life using shared parental leave. However, as few as 5 per cent of those who are eligible actually do this. In other countries, for example Sweden and Finland, large blocks of paternity leave are the norm.

When it comes to the influence of fathers on future stress, there is less evidence than there is for mothers, but plenty of research has been done, and it all points towards a significant impact. A string of studies have shown that children with engaged, warm fathers have lower cortisol levels than those without. This is not just about the early years – the same effect is shown repeatedly in adolescents. In contrast, a father who is depressed after a baby is born – postnatal depression can also affect men, with some estimates saying up to 1 in 10 fathers is affected – is linked with not just future behavioural issues but stress-connected physical ailments like abdominal pain. One study found a particular association between fathers who use physical coercion, such as spanking or slapping, and elevated cortisol in children's hair samples.[21]

There is, however, an even bigger lesson lurking in the background, one that goes well beyond the endless debates about father or mothers, childcare or stay-at-home caregiver. A lot of this is shaped by significantly wider factors than choice or parenting methods. One is the fairly obvious fact that no one begins their parenting experience as a blank slate. Repeated studies, not just in people but also in animals as varied as rats and apes, has shown that one of the most significant predictors of how someone will parent is the way they were parented themselves. Once again, this is not an inevitable determinant. Having a less-than-ideal parental figure does not mean someone will be the same. But it is likely to play a role.

Also, as with more or less everything else connected to stress, income and social status plays its part. A long-term British study found that one of the strongest predictors of low birth weight, itself one of the most significant indicators of future stress and poor health, was socioeconomic status.[22] In what takes us into even more sensitive territory, observation studies of infants with their parents have concluded that a greater level of parental education and a higher income tends to correlate with more stimulating engagement with the child.[23]

Along with all the usual caveats about this being a case of broad-brush averages, there is also research suggesting the correlation can sometimes go the other way. An intriguing recent US study sought to work out how parents could best help their children with an artificially-created stressful situation, in this case a presentation about themselves to a hypothetical new teacher. The children, aged nine to eleven, had a parent with them who was simply told to 'provide support to your child in any way you find useful'. Children whose parents had a degree were found to have notably higher cortisol levels by the end of the presentation than those whose parents did not. The researchers surmised that parents who are more highly educated might place emphasis on the child doing 'well' in the presentation, while the others gave less pressurized support and comfort.[24]

Once again, there is no one-size-fits-all answer, just a succession of scattered clues to be interpreted and somehow fitted into the existing clutter and confusion of our lives. Donald Winnicott was right: trying to be the perfect father, mother, or any other variety of childhood caregiver, will see you very much on a hiding to nothing.

After this focus on childhood health outcomes, and the decades of research zeroing-in on mothers, it is worth reflecting on the ways that women in particular are affected by stress. To reiterate another theme of this book, it is not always a level playing field.

To begin with, study after study has shown that women, on average, experience greater levels of chronic stress than men. This is the product of a very long list of factors, including ingrained discrimination, particularly in work, and societal pressures, some related to appearance and weight. None of this is to suggest that men do not face many similar pressures, or to diminish the impact of these. It is not a contest.

Added to this are potential stressors from women's and men's differing responsibilities. Many decades of studies have shown that, on average, even when both partners work, women tend to take greater responsibility not just for domestic and child-related tasks, but for general 'life administration'. This takes a toll. Pioneering research by a Swedish psychologist called Marianne Frankenhaeuser in the 1980s showed that while men and women had similar levels of stress while at work, when they returned home the men's physical stress indicators would fall swiftly, whereas for women they would generally take much longer to drop, or in some cases they would rise even more.[25]

It is perhaps no surprise that when men and women are asked about their stress, women tend to report higher amounts. The American Psychological Association's annual study of stress across the US, which we mentioned in Chapter 5, shows that when asked for their stress levels on a scale of one to ten, the female average was 5.3, against 4.9 for men. Significantly more women than men placed their levels of stress as being eight or above.[26]

All this has physical implications. One of the starkest gender differences in health is that while women live longer than men, on average, their rate of chronic ailments is much higher. One study went through thirty different such conditions, everything from joint pain to intestinal troubles, and found that 90 per cent of them are more common in women. Another huge research project on the prevalence of chronic pain, which questioned 85,000 people, found that women were more likely to experience pain than men in every one of the seventeen countries studied.[27]

This so-called female–male health–survival paradox is not entirely caused by stress. Part of the problem appears to be a medical tilt towards focusing on lethal conditions rather than debilitating ones, and also the well-chronicled tendency for doctors to neglect illnesses faced predominantly or entirely by women, many of them linked to menstruation and their wider reproductive systems, whether they have children or not. But it is notable how many of them are strongly linked to stress.

One good example is fibromyalgia, a long-term condition which causes widespread musculoskeletal pain and tenderness, as well as fatigue and a difficulty in concentrating known as 'fibro fog'. This has a well-documented tendency to begin or flare up in response to stress. One very recent study put the proportion of diagnosed fibromyalgia sufferers who are women as between 80 and 96 per cent.[28] And with an estimated 2 million people affected by it in the UK alone, this is not a small problem.

Research into stress as it affects women can sometimes feel like we are still stuck in the Hans Selye era of it being seen as a problem for male business executives. Gail Kinman, the professor of occupational health psychology who we heard from in Chapter 5, says part of this is a legacy from decades of academic study. 'For quite a long time, pretty much all research in psychology in general was done with men,' she says. 'And not just men, but young, white, middle-class American students. It was then extrapolated out to everybody else. Some of the early research didn't use humans at all – it was rats and mice. But never women.'

Another difficulty in assessing gender differences in stress is that a good deal of them can be hidden. To return to Joeli Brearley, whose abrupt loss of work began this chapter: her campaign group, Pregnant Then Screwed, began as a website where women could tell their own, similar stories, anonymously if needed. Many of these, it turned out, were being recounted for the very first time. Brearley says that as well as being amazed to learn how many women had gone through experiences like hers, another revelation was the high proportion who were not able to discuss what happened openly, because the company concerned had paid them off with the addition of a so-called non-disclosure agreement, or NDA. Signing this would often bring more money than they would be likely to get awarded by an industrial tribunal, and without the risk. But it also meant that if they told anyone about their experiences, they could be sued.

'An NDA literally tells you that you're only allowed to speak to your lawyer and your spouse about it,' Brearley says. 'Every woman I've spoken to who signed one regrets it, because it sort of sits within like a dark secret. When you work in another company, colleagues become friends, and you can't even tell *them* what happened in your last job. You can't say, "They screwed me over, they treated me really appallingly. And that's why I had to leave." It's layers of lies, when it was something really traumatic that happened to them. For the employer, they just pay a sum of money and don't think about it again.'

Brearley says the entire experience often creates a huge amount of stress, at a time when women are, much as she was, being urged to avoid this: 'I've spoken to lots of women who are essentially teaching themselves employment law while caring for a new baby on maternity leave. It's one thing having to think about the high rates of postnatal depression without trying to learn employment law in a few months.'

Brearley sees herself as one of the luckier ones. As well as being healthy, her son was not even born small. Setting up Pregnant Then Screwed has helped her deal with her feelings to the extent that she no longer feels anger towards the woman who dismissed her for being pregnant.

This is an uplifting end to a difficult story. Not everyone, however, gets the chance to banish their demons in such a cathartic way. As we have seen in this chapter, stress in pregnancy, infancy and early childhood, whether affecting a parent, carer or child, can generate consequences lasting not just decades, but generations.

Such an endless parade of research and experience can feel almost exhausting, even demoralizing. Stress, as we have seen in these past nine chapters, is inescapable. How, then, can you mitigate it? It is to this, finally, that we move next.

CHAPTER 10

Routes Out of Stress

You could perhaps argue that a chapter offering tips on how to cope with stress risks falling somewhere between a near-impossibility and an outright con. As we have seen repeatedly throughout the book, stress and its impacts are both highly individualized and, in the majority of instances, caused by things well beyond anyone's personal control. It's possible that the most honest if disheartening tip for someone who is stressed and wants to know how to stop it would be: don't start from here.

If at this point you are tempted to flick straight to the final chapter in the hope of finding something cheerier, don't despair. As we are about to explain, it would also be misleading to suggest nothing can be done.

One of the curiosities of stress is that its very slipperiness – the way it presents such a broad front in its impact on humans – also gives lots of ingress points when fighting back. Even if the cause of your stress can seem intractable, there are often ways to mitigate it, or at the very least to try to limit some of the physical consequences. There isn't always a way out. But more often than not, something can be done. And often, the first step can just be to realize that you are stressed. As ever with the subject, even this initial self-knowledge and acceptance depends hugely on the context.

Let us illustrate this with a pair of academic studies which, even by the standards of the often inventive research into stress that we have seen across this book, were pretty distinctive.

The first took place in 1977 and involved the famed Austrian conductor Herbert von Karajan. Organized by his compatriot, the psychiatrist Gerhart Harrer – who, like von Karajan, had a very successful post-war career despite some troublingly close links to the Nazi regime – it saw the conductor wired up to a series of heart and skin monitors as he listened to a recording of Beethoven's *'Leonore' Overture No.3*, before later conducting the same piece with the Berlin Philharmonic, the orchestra he led for thirty-four years. Finally, von Karajan was rigged up once more as he flew his own small plane through a series of somewhat risky manoeuvres.

Von Karajan's body responded strongly to the same particularly rousing sections of the Beethoven piece, both when he was listening and conducting, although understandably the effect was stronger when he was leading the orchestra. But interestingly, his heart rate when conducting the orchestra was also significantly higher than when he was flying, even when the latter involved him approaching the runway to land before suddenly pulling up and regaining altitude, on one occasion deliberately putting the plane into a roll as he climbed.[1]

Just over twenty years later, academic research looked once again at the orchestral world, but from another perspective. Headed by the renowned expert on stress, Seymour Levine, the co-author was his son, Robert, who happened to be the principal violinist of the Milwaukee Symphony Orchestra. As you can guess from the title of the eventual paper, 'Why they're not smiling: stress and discontent in the orchestra workplace', this argued that despite being paid to pursue what was presumably their lifelong passion, many orchestral players were often stressed. Why? One element was the anxiety of having to perform perfectly and be constantly measured against their colleagues. Another reason reintroduces a key concept from earlier in the book: control.

As explained at length by the two Levines, orchestras are somewhere between a patriarchy and an outright dictatorship, led by the omniscient figure of the conductor, who is generally addressed as 'Maestro' (they added: 'This title may be dropped if the conductor is sufficiently young or doesn't speak with an accent.') Orchestral musicians are, the study noted, very clearly experts themselves, not children. Nonetheless, an ensemble of up to a hundred musicians cannot run themselves, and so they must give up any autonomy: 'They do not control when the music starts, when the music ends, or how the music goes. They don't even have the authority to leave the stage to attend to personal needs. They are, in essence, rats in a maze, at the whim of the god with the baton.' It was no surprise, the paper said, to find that in their leisure time, orchestral musicians tend to dislike team sports, preferring more individual hobbies.[2]

What do these two closely linked and yet very different pieces of research tell us? A few things, one of which returns us to almost the very first point of this book. Stress cannot be measured neutrally, or placed in a formal league table. Not only is it entirely subjective in its impact, but it can mean several very different things at the same time – and not all of them necessarily bad.

Conducting music, to von Karajan, was very clearly something which, by standard physiological gauges, created turmoil in his body. There would have been some very real stress – not least that no one wants to mess up in front of a hundred underlings who, if the Levines' study is to be believed, possibly hold you in mild contempt anyway. But this was also a form of exhilaration, the same sort of intoxicating rush of hormones experienced by an Olympic diver as they are propelled upward by the springboard, or an actor when they step onto the stage.

Such a response is largely predicated on control. Whether waving his baton or flying his plane, von Karajan was someone with very high social and professional status who had chosen to do these particular things and could equally have not done them. By contrast, as a violinist, let alone a warehouse worker like Anna from Chapter 5, you have pretty much no say in matters beyond deciding to quit your job. This means the hormonal surge and other bodily responses might be broadly the same in physiological terms, but they could affect you in a completely different way.

All this is a slightly convoluted way to introduce a note of caution for this chapter: in trying to find ways to cope with stress, it all depends on the circumstances. Also, much as stress affects people's bodies very differently, it is the same when it comes to its solutions. Yoga, mindfulness or running might help alleviate it in some people, but for many others it might not. As one study author put it, in a reference to the origins of the word 'stress' from materials science, 'The engineer can have confidence in a foreseeable relationship between stressor and stress; one steel girder will behave much like the next. This is not the case for human stress.'[3] So, if you have turned immediately to this chapter in the hope of seeing a simple list of Ten Ways to Beat Stress, that is not what you will find. There are no all-purpose, works-for-everyone solutions. But there are answers, of a sort.

Kate's story

Kate was referred to Richard's clinic by a gynaecologist because of her irregular periods. There were also concerns about her apparently fluctuating weight, even though her BMI was well within normal bounds. Finally, there was a request to measure her blood glucose and insulin resistance in case these were elevated. They were not. All these worries and demands, it should be mentioned, were relayed not by Kate, but by her mother, who booked the appointment on her behalf and came along.

Kate, who was nineteen at the time, stayed largely silent. Once or twice, when she did start to explain a point, her mother would talk over her. When the pair were told that Kate's BMI and body composition readings were entirely standard for her age, the mother intervened again, talking about portion sizes and how she always prepared healthy meals for her daughter. Kate was very obviously much loved. She was also in many ways materially and socially privileged. Her family was relatively well-off, she had done well at school and was taking a year off before going to university. But in other ways, she was as trapped as a violinist in an orchestra.

Kate only came to the clinic once, so there is no update, happy or otherwise, to relay. But what her story does illustrate is that no one is immune from stress. Her early years were almost certainly free of family worries about bills, or the threat of being evicted. Her parents both had well-paid, professional jobs. Nonetheless, her background seemed likely to set her on a course for elevated cortisol and all the problems that come with that.

The slightly contradictory point which should also be noted is that the same epidemiological statistics which make Kate a possible candidate for future type 2 diabetes also presents a very eloquent case for her being something of an exception. While everyone faces stress, it is an inescapable fact that being financially and professionally secure insulates you from some of the most common and chronic pressures.

The sheer remorselessness of the societal factors behind public health were eloquently highlighted by a British academic called David Gordon, an expert on poverty, who compiled a set of 'alternative tips' for good health, using his years of research to gently mock the sorts of lists you see in lifestyle magazines and government campaigns. In place of exhortations like 'Don't smoke', 'Eat plenty of fruit and vegetables' and 'Keep physically active', he had 'Don't be poor', 'Don't live in a deprived area' and 'Don't be disabled or have a disabled child.' Rather than advising people to manage stress by relaxing where possible, Gordon put 'Don't work in a stressful, low-paid, manual job.'[4]

All this is, very obviously, impossible. But at the same time, while Kate was neither poor nor disabled, it would have been equally useless to offer her the stress-based advice of 'Try to have different parents.' That's the thing with stress: several factors can be true at the same time.

When it comes to possible solutions, one thing to consider is the almost paradoxical notion that if a stressor is inescapable, it can sometimes be better to simply not try to find a way out, but instead to detach yourself from it. This was illustrated in a fascinating study of Black teenagers growing up in a disadvantaged part of Chicago, which found that they tended to cope with the range of pressures in one of two broad ways: cognitive engagement with the stressor, as a means to try and resolve it; or what the study termed 'avoidance and distraction'. When it came to stresses like school, the first approach seemed to work better. But for worries about violence, whether from the police or local gangs, those who were able to disengage tended to have better mental outcomes, even though the researchers noted that this tactic was often difficult to achieve.[5]

Another potential approach, if tackling the origin of the stress appears impossible, is to instead focus on the symptoms, notably physical ones. Leaving a pressured job might be financially impossible, while a predisposition to high cortisol which was set in infancy is tricky to reset, even with something like long-term therapy. But if the stress manifests in the body as, say, insulin resistance, this is often more receptive to potential intervention, whether through a changed diet or more physical activity, or in some cases medication.

Having warned in Chapter 6 about guilt over diet and weight, it is now time to sound the same alarm about exercise and fitness. Pretty much everyone knows that being more active will, in almost any circumstances, be good for their health. But at the same time, a lot of people don't manage it. Around 4 in 10 British adults are sufficiently inactive that their long-term health is at risk, irrespective of whether or not they are stressed, a statistic which is broadly typical by global standards. This is not caused by a mass outbreak of laziness. It is simply that the world around us has changed over recent decades such that inactivity is the norm – everything from the replacement of manual work with desk jobs, to towns and cities built around cars. It is the physical equivalent of an obesogenic environment, and closely linked to it. Unhealthy choices become the default. This is all the more the case if you have a disability. If choosing physical movement is difficult even if you are able-bodied, it can at times be almost impossible if you have a disability.

Once everyday exertion is effectively banished, for many people the only option is formal exercise, which uses up time they might not have and requires motivation which can be difficult to maintain. Hence statistics showing that 10 per cent of gym memberships are not used, while more than half of British adults never take part in any type of sport.

This is a subject largely outside the remit of this book, but it's worth remembering two things. One is that guilt won't help at all, and can contribute to experiencing even more stress. The other is that if you can find a way to build physical movement into your everyday life then there is, statistically, a greater chance it will stick. Something like walking or cycling for your commute is what public health experts call 'incidental activity', just another part of your existing routine. This is distinct from 'discretionary time', those precious leisure hours where you could be with your family or friends, or watching TV with a glass of wine, rather than working up a sweat on a gym treadmill.

But if you do manage to become more physically active, however you manage it, then the benefits are pretty much immediate and at times not far short of miraculous.

The man who invented exercise

Unlikely as it might sound, as recently as the 1950s many scientists believed that strenuous exercise was actually something of a health risk, particularly for the heart. One man changed that: the extraordinary and largely unknown Jerry Morris.

Born into poverty in Glasgow to Jewish immigrant parents who had fled what is now Belarus, Morris became an epidemiologist, a doctor who looks at population-wide health trends. Asked to examine why heart attack rates were rising in post-war Britain, Morris studied the health records from thousands of London public transport workers. He spotted that bus conductors, who were on their feet and up and down stairs all day collecting tickets, had notably lower heart disease rates than their colleagues who drove the vehicles. After going through all the possibilities, he worked out that this must be due to their activity levels.

> Morris's findings, published in a 1953 edition of *The Lancet*,[6] prompted a notably hostile reaction, with many people deeply reluctant to believe that a desk job, one of the main aspirations of the period, could actually be bad for you.
>
> They were mistaken, and a mass of subsequent studies, many also by Morris, proved the case. Morris, who always walked up the stairs to his office and took every other opportunity he could to be active, lived to be ninety-nine, having spent decades trying to persuade successive British governments to help people live more active lives, with notably limited success.

Stress, as we have seen, can create or exacerbate a long list of ailments. In more or less every instance, being more active helps to alleviate them. This appears to be particularly so with metabolic and inflammatory disorders such as type 2 diabetes. We saw in the first chapter how Ruth's diabetes effectively went into remission after she got a dog and began to swim. The exercise does not have to be strenuous. Studies have shown that even walking for thirty minutes a day cuts the risks associated with type 2 diabetes by 50 per cent on average. Such is the impact of activity on diabetes that one piece of Richard's work showed that diabetic risk is lessened in sedentary rodents who receive a blood transfusion from a well-exercised one.[7]

There are reams of studies illustrating how activity and exercise greatly reduces people's risk of heart disease, high blood pressure and strokes. It also helps alleviate depression and anxiety, makes you sleep better and improves your cognitive performance. Newer studies have shown it can even help reverse non-alcoholic fatty liver disease. One of the most famous pieces of research, carried out in Denmark, tracked around 30,000 randomly selected people of all ages over a period of fifteen years. It found that even when all other demographic, social and lifestyle factors were taken into account, people who commuted by bike were 40 per cent less likely to have died over the study period than those who did not. From any cause.[8]

A lot of recent focus has been on how this effect happens at a cellular level, with particular attention given to something called 'tissue crosstalk', also known as 'bone-muscle crosstalk'. When stimulated by exercise, the process prompts an endocrine response involving proteins including myokines, which we encountered in Chapter 3, and another type of protein called osteokines, which are vital for bone homeostasis. Yet another relevant protein is the awkwardly-named brain-derived neurotrophic factor (BDNF). This is a key player in learning and memory, and is also heavily involved in alleviating stress. Being more active appears to stimulate their collaborative work.

One obvious caveat with exerting yourself to relieve stress is to be wary about large amounts of very intense exercise, something which, as we have seen, can stimulate the cortisol response all over again. The key seems to be to keep the exertion below about 60 per cent of your aerobic capacity – you're definitely working hard, but not to exhaustion.

For people without flashy exercise watches and heart-rate zone charts, how can you tell when you're pushing things too far? One thing to watch out for seems to be the tempo of the music you listen to. Research has indicated that this is the key factor in determining exertion rates, more so than whether you actually like the song, or even the style of music. One study saw a group of people told to do their 'normal' workout on stationary bikes to the accompaniment of music of different genres and tempos. The quicker the beat, the faster and more vigorously they cycled, whether the music was rock, country or polka. Yes, polka.[9]

This is not a hard-and-fast rule, simply a factor to be aware of. Plenty of people can exercise at relentless intensity without a hint of longer-term cortisol build-up. Such exertion can even, some studies have shown, help people cope better with an immediately stressful situation. One experiment involved submitting a group of young men to the forbidding Trier Social Stress Test, as described in Chapter 3. It found that those who preceded it with a vigorous run on a treadmill had lower overall cortisol levels and a quicker return to baseline levels than those who did a light or moderate workout.[10]

If that wasn't confusing enough already, other research has argued that when it comes to some markers for stress, exercise has to hit some level of duration to make a real difference. A Finnish team took a cohort of thousands of people and measured what is known as C-reactive protein, or CRP, elevated levels of which are strongly linked to a host of inflammation-based ailments. They found that those who regularly commuted by bike tended to have lower CRP concentrations, but that this effect only seemed to really take effect when people cycled at least forty-five minutes a day.[11]

By now, you might be wondering whether to block-book a series of high-intensity exercise classes, go for a long walk or bike ride, or just stay at home entirely. The big picture is that exercise or other types of exertion will almost always help with stress, but that you need to listen to your body. It is also less likely to help if it becomes just yet another onerous, guilt-inducing chore. Similarly, exercise you love can be relaxing.

Regardless of how potent, exercise and physical movement are among the many ways to try to combat stress and its repercussions. And so, in what might seem a flagrant breach of our self-imposed 'no lists' rule for this book, we shall, well, list a few others. But rest assured: these are ideas, not recommendations. What actually works could be different for almost everyone.

Touch

As we saw in the last chapter, with everyone from Romanian orphans to rat pups, physical touch from a mother, father or other caregiver is one of the fundamentals to how our response to stress is established in infancy. The good news is that it also seems to work as a means to relieve stress whatever stage of life you are at.

Over the years there have been endless studies showing that

owning a pet can mitigate stress and make people less likely to see a doctor. This is particularly the case with dogs, and particularly for older owners, most likely in part because having a dog obliges you to leave the house and go for a walk, and often to interact with other people. Dogs and other pets are also generally very soothing to stroke. But, it turns out, an animal doesn't have to be fluffy for this to happen.

One very innovative study saw a group of Israeli university students and staff presented with a task which was, if anything, even more sadistic than the Trier stress test's mock presentation to a roomful of blank-faced scientists. When each volunteer arrived, a researcher uncovered a glass jar containing a large tarantula and breezily told them they would be assigned either to a group which would just look at the spider or to one that would be asked to hold it. After the researcher left the room with the excuse of fetching something, the subjects were randomly handed one of four things: a rabbit, a turtle, a toy rabbit or a toy turtle. They were simply told to 'hold and pet it for a while'. At various points they were asked questions for a standardized test on their feelings of stress and anxiety.

The findings were striking. As you might expect, people felt notably more soothed after petting one of the real animals rather than the toys, but there was no discernible difference between the rabbit and the turtle, or between their toy equivalents. It was, the researchers concluded, the 'quality of being alive rather than the texture of the object that produced the effect'. The same thing happened whether or not people described themselves as animal lovers. And in case you were wondering: no, the test subjects never had to hold the tarantula. That was just a ruse.[12]

The effect animals have goes beyond touch – just being in a room with them can prove relaxing. Another study, this time in the US, put children aged three to six through a doctor's examination involving a stethoscope and various other tests, once with a beagle standing near them, once without. As measured by blood pressure and heart rate, the presence of the dog seemed to make the children considerably less stressed.[13]

Pets, obviously, are not an entirely straightforward solution to stress even if you love animals, given that they come with obligations – not just walks and company for dogs, but what can be expensive vet bills. Luckily, touch works in other ways – even, it seems, when it is self-administered. A recent experiment at a German university saw 150 volunteers put through the Trier Social Stress Test – this time they were told to present a pitch for their dream job – and have their cortisol levels tested. As ever, they were split into three groups. Before the test, one received a 20-second hug from one of the research assistants; another was told to touch or stroke themselves in a way that felt comfortable; the third did neither. The results? Those who were hugged had notably lower cortisol levels than the people who received no touch at all, but so did the people who self-soothed.[14]

Company

This is an area just as well-researched as touch, but it can be significantly harder to fix. Decades of studies have demonstrated that much as feeling lonely or isolated is a major indicator of stress, having social support and connectedness very much helps to relieve it.

One of the most famous pieces of research into the subject was carried out in the mid-1970s by Michael Marmot, the British expert on health inequalities who we have encountered at various points across the book. He examined rates of heart disease among more than 4,000 Americans of Japanese ancestry, trying to work out why their rates of heart disease were notably higher than those of people in Japan.

He found that even when other lifestyle and health factors were taken into account, the more people were exposed to traditional Japanese values, the lower their heart disease levels, something the study attributed to the Japanese cultural emphasis on group cohesion. The effect was striking: Japanese Americans who had most assimilated into US ways of living had heart disease levels between three and five times higher than those who had done so the least.[15]

Understandably, there has been a mass of studies about stress and loneliness based around Covid lockdowns, with some interesting results. One joint UK–US project found that when it came to alleviating stress from the pandemic, what mattered was not the size of the household people were living with, but the quality of the relationships, and that living with a spouse or partner appeared particularly useful in buffering the strains.

Psychotherapy

This one word covers a realm of styles and methods, and the field is equally broad when it comes to addressing stress. It is also a deeply personal endeavour. What works for one person will not necessarily work for another. If you think it might help you, it's possibly worth first speaking to a practitioner, a professional body or a knowledgeable friend. Some people find it useful to have an introductory session with more than one therapist, given the importance of the personal connection.

As an overview, there are a few general ways to try to assist with stress through therapy, with plenty of studies backing the effectiveness of them all, albeit with the caveat that a lot depends on the person and the situation.

The first is so-called cognitive behavioural therapy, or CBT, which tends to be shorter-term and more directly results-focused. Someone might try CBT, for example, to try to tackle a particular source of stress and its impact, for example becoming panicked before work meetings.

Then there is more traditional therapy, which like CBT is also generally a single fifty-minute session per week, although here, some people go twice a week, or even more often (particularly in the more traditional, Freudian world). Like CBT, this can be short-term, perhaps for twelve weeks, or it can be open-ended. Longer-term therapy can be particularly good at helping people understand the wider reasons why certain stresses affect them, given the links to childhood or infancy.

When set out in this way, psychotherapy can sound a bit formless, even woolly, but many people are surprised at how incisive it proves. A therapist is not a life coach, suggesting ideas or solutions. If you think of the process as a walk through unfamiliar countryside in the dusk, a therapist is not a guide with a map, just someone who can occasionally shine a torch so you can see your own way more clearly. Even if there are stressful aspects of your life which you cannot immediately change, simply understanding them better can make a major difference.

Sleep

Much like social connections, this has the slight risk of being filed under 'Pointing out the obvious' and 'I would if I could'. Also, even more than with many areas of stress, it is difficult to disentangle what comes first. As we saw in Chapter 3, sleep deprivation and sleep disruption can affect the HPA axis. This is particularly the case given the way that natural cortisol concentrations are so tied to the sleep cycle, reaching a peak just before we would normally wake up and then gradually falling across the day. But also, stress is a very obvious source of disrupted sleep in the first place.

There is also a strong association between poor sleep patterns and insulin resistance, weight gain and, possibly, type 2 diabetes. Studies have shown that even in healthy people, a lack of sleep can cause a 30 per cent drop in insulin signalling, the molecular-level process by which insulin goes about its work, and can create insulin resistance in fat cells. Very new research suggests that this fat-specific insulin resistance could be the early starting point for the development of type 2 diabetes.[16]

A recent meta-study into sleep and cortisol levels found relatively limited amounts of direct research into the specifics of this stress–sleep mechanism, but did uncover one apparent constant: more physical activity is associated not only with lower cortisol concentrations, but also with better sleep. Once again, it seems to be a magic cure.[17]

How to improve your sleep is a subject almost as complex and argued-over as stress itself, with very nearly as many 'how to' books penned on the subject. As such, offering a few tips would barely scratch the surface. The answer is likely to be slightly different for everyone. Additionally, many of the most common suggestions (keep a set routine, have a calm, quiet bedroom), in yet another echo of stress, are often beyond someone's control.

Caffeine

This merits a separate heading from sleep because it has a stress-related effect that goes beyond its more well-known tendency to keep you awake.

Caffeine is a potent stimulator of bodily glucose uptake, so much so that it is sometimes used in laboratory cell-culture experiments to understand the mechanisms which regulate how cells take up sugar. This is mainly due to caffeine's ability to increase intracellular calcium levels, which provoke something called the AMP-activated protein kinase (AMPK) pathway into action. This has a central role in regulating cellular energy homeostasis and appears to be behind the apparent correlation between caffeine intake and insulin resistance in non-diabetic people, with some studies demonstrating it can worsen people's scores on the test for insulin resistance.

Caffeine can also directly increase cortisol secretion by elevating the production of adrenocorticotropin hormone (ACTH), the substance which prompts the pituitary gland to produce cortisol. Caffeine intake is also linked with increased blood pressure and heart rate, two physiological responses regulated by cortisol. Thus, having caffeine when you're already stressed could further elevate your cortisol.

This is very much not a recommendation to stop drinking coffee, not least if giving up your morning latte or Americano might feel, well, stressful. This is just a note of the possible impacts. It's worth remembering that while caffeine does increase blood pressure, if you're not otherwise stressed, the effect is short-lived.

Diet

This is not about 'diet' in the sense of tips for weight loss, but about foods which seem to have stress-reducing properties. There is, however, one thing to consider first: ways to eat, which seems to combat one of the major knock-on physical symptoms of stress. An increasing amount of evidence indicates that intermittent fasting – or its close cousin, time-restricted eating – can have a real impact on insulin resistance.

Intermittent fasting has various forms, such as eating every other day, or five days out of seven – the so-called 5:2 approach. With time-restricted eating, the idea is to keep all food intake within a window of around eight hours, for example by missing breakfast and not eating after 8 p.m. Both have recently become popular as potential weight-loss methods, but the research so far is more conclusive about the effect they appear to have on insulin resistance. A series of studies have shown that both techniques tend to boost insulin sensitivity, as well as improving how the body metabolizes fats. They can even reduce blood pressure. All this is independent from any effect from simply losing weight.

So, how does it work? A long gap between meals appears to allow the body to have, in simple terms, a bit of a break, helping insulin levels to fall, which assists with homeostasis.

When it comes to *what* to eat, rather than *when*, research has shown that the so-called Mediterranean diet, based on lots of vegetables, fruit, whole grains and olive oil, as well as fish but minimal meat, can dampen the stress response in both human teenagers and long-tailed macaques – groups which some parents may think share a few similarities. The benefits of this diet can, however, take time to manifest. In the research, the macaques were fed a Mediterranean diet for thirty-one months – nine years in human terms.[18] A variant on the research, involving around 300 staff at an Israeli nuclear facility, tried people on something called the Green Mediterranean diet, involving even more vegetables, as well as teas and supplements rich in polyphenols, which are found in a variety of foods and known for their anti-inflammatory properties. After six months, waking cortisol levels were roughly similar between the three different groups: normal diet, Mediterranean and Green Mediterranean. But after eighteen months, the Mediterranean eaters saw their cortisol levels drop, while the Green Mediterranean group experienced an even greater fall.[19]

If drinking a shake made from *Wolffia globosa*, a polyphenol-rich type of Asian duckweed, is not necessarily your thing, there is always chocolate – but not just any chocolate. One test showed that four weeks of daily consumption of a polyphenol-heavy dark chocolate lowered people's saliva cortisol, while standard dark chocolate did not.[20] How does this happen? It seems to be something to do with the ability of some polyphenols to reduce the potency of an enzyme called 11beta-hydroxysteroid dehydrogenase, which converts inactive cortisone into active cortisol. The same effect has been observed in tests using other polyphenol-heavy substances such as extracts from *Hibiscus sabdariffa*, a subtropical variety of the hibiscus plant, native to Africa.

Mindfulness, yoga and aromatherapy

This might be a good moment to reiterate that this is a list of things which have been shown to help some people. It is not a directive. Some of the ideas below, like inhaling lavender oil or trying 'laughter yoga', could prompt feelings of scepticism, even annoyance, in certain readers. That is not a failing. But if you are tempted, the evidence for such interventions is pretty strong. This is also the case for mindfulness, a type of meditation in which people try to focus very strongly on being in the here-and-now.

One of the more recent studies tested out a two-month mindfulness programme on what might seem an unpromising cohort: a hundred or so police officers in the US Midwest. But the scheme, which provided lessons in mindfulness and encouraged the officers to practise it for twenty minutes a day, recorded notably lower waking cortisol after three months in those who did this, compared to a control group who did not; they also slept better.[21]

One of the good things about mindfulness as a stress intervention, if you do feel it might work for you, is the relatively short amount of time it takes to do and the many ways you can learn it, including online courses and a wealth of apps.

Yoga has a similarly good record, with meta-studies collating various research projects tending to conclude that it successfully mitigates stress symptoms, albeit with some uncertainty as to how this happens. This can happen even when the stress is very deep-seated, as with one test which found that a ten-week yoga programme significantly improved both cortisol levels and sleep for a group of US military veterans who had experienced post-traumatic stress disorder.[22]

A different study, one based in Germany, took a group of volunteers through, yet again, the Trier Social Stress Test, with some of these preceding it with what is called 'laughter yoga', where yoga exercises are mixed with laughter. Those who took part had lower levels of cortisol following the stress test than those who didn't.[23]

Another option which some might initially view as New Age nonsense, but which is backed by proper evidence, is aromatherapy. Simply inhaling a diluted essence of lavender was shown to reduce both perceived anxiety and cortisol concentrations for people facing the very obviously stressful prospect of open-heart surgery.[24] Other aromas, including cedarwood and vetiver, have also been shown to curb cortisol levels, in stressed rats.[25]

Reducing screen time

Spending a lot of time staring at phones, tablets or laptops is often mentioned in relation to stress – and yes, there are studies linking the two. However, no one has yet concluded whether this is a causal relationship, or just correlative. Long periods of screen time are also connected to worse sleep and lower physical activity levels, which have their own impact on stress. It could be that these are the significant factors; as yet, we don't know.

The best advice here would be to listen to your body and try to be sensible, however imperfect a recommendation that might seem. If you find it hard to sleep after staring at a phone or tablet in bed, try to leave devices in another room. In parallel with the still-developing literature on screen use and stress is the yet-more-contested study of stress induced by social media. Once again, the best idea is to listen to yourself: if you feel edgy after an hour of doom-scrolling the news, have a think about whether it's something you really want to do. But equally, if it's a useful way to relax, don't feel guilty about it.

Listening to music

While this idea has been studied for many more decades than the impact of screen time, the conclusions are only slightly more definitive. Various studies have suggested that music that is more soothing, in particular, can have a stress-alleviating impact. But it all depends on context.

One of the biggest variables is choice. One person might find that some inoffensive, saxophone-led light jazz is the perfect tonic for their cortisol levels; another might find it hugely irritating, especially when it is being played to them without any say. Once again, control can be key.

All that said, there is some evidence that certain types of music are more stress-relieving than others. One US study found that even when a group of college students were allowed to select their own music, those who picked heavy metal showed less sign of stress relief then the ones who listened to a classical composition.

How do this book's authors cope with stress?

Peter: Perhaps a bit boringly, my main way to try to mitigate stress is physical movement. Some of this is formal exercise but the bulk is cycling around London, where I live, for transport. Lots of people might, very understandably, view riding a bike in a big city as a stressful experience in itself. But I find it almost meditative – at least most of the time. As a stress reliever it has the added bonus of almost always getting me to my destination more or less exactly when I expected. More generally, I had several years of psychotherapy in the past, not to address any particular issue but to help me understand a few wider things in my life. I can't definitively say if it made me less stressed, but it certainly gave me a lot of context. And while my day job as a politics journalist can be fairly relentless, I'm lucky to have very supportive, empathic and fun colleagues. Sadly, these cannot be prescribed on the NHS.

Richard: I deal with stress in many ways. I have always run; it allows me to switch off from the world and take time out for myself. Importantly, I do this to music that either calms me or gets me moving faster, depending on my mood. I enjoy cooking and find myself unwinding most evenings torturing some very lovely ingredients into a mess on my plate. But at the heart of how I deal with my own stress is something that most find difficult to do. This is forgiveness. It's hard to let the past go, particularly if someone has hurt you emotionally or physically. But I worked out that if I didn't find forgiveness, then the people that get hurt the most are those closest to you. Then there is the last route I use to de-stress: my son. I think about his little warm smile and his energy for life. To use a quote from a good friend, it's hard to 'sweat the small stuff' when I have his face pictured in my head.

Lessons from animals

In the near-century since Hans Selye introduced the modern era of stress with his clumsily handled mice, a vast amount of research has been based around animals of more or less every sort. Much of this has involved rats (fast to grow; notably more intelligent than mice), and a great variety of monkeys and apes. Other tests have looked at the stress response in oysters, salmon, deer spooked by exposure to human visitors, and even the Chinese three-keeled pond turtle. One very recent study from Slovakia tried to find out if racehorses were stressed by any aspects of their regime, including training, jumps and transportation between events. Horses are not very good at taking standard saliva cortisol tests, so the ingenious research team attached tampons to long pieces of string, allowed the horses to chew on them for a while, and then pulled them out. The conclusions? Apart from a very slight cortisol reaction to being transported, the horses seemed to quite enjoy it all.[26]

While animal research has helped with many breakthroughs in stress research, there is one very obvious difference with humans. Animals react to acute stress, they can also experience chronic stress – but they do not repeatedly trigger their HPA axis simply by anticipating or considering long-term or speculative pressures. People, of course, do this a lot.

Robert Sapolsky, the famous American biologist who has spent two decades studying stress in a troop of Kenyan baboons and was quoted in Chapter 5, once described, in his typically playful way, how stress is both universal across vertebrate animals and unique in its effect on people: 'It is startling to realise that a vast length of time ago, while evading a predator or pursuing a prey, a dinosaur secreted glucocorticoids. Despite this conservatism and antiquity of the adrenocortical stress response, a point must be made, however – no dinosaur ever worried itself sick from perseverating on the absurd idea that an asteroid might strike Earth.'[27]

Sapolsky's long period in the Serengeti region, in which he would devise ever-more cunning ruses to be able to tranquillize the wily baboons so he could test their cortisol levels, taught him many lessons which are highly relevant to the human condition. His years of work have showed that, much as with people, being a subordinate baboon in the troop, and thus subject to the whims of more physically powerful and better socially-connected animals, exacted a greater psychological and physiological price than being dominant. This is the case, at least, when the hierarchy was stable; when there was sudden social flux for whatever reason, cortisol levels soared in the baboons seeking to fight, intimidate and otherwise scheme their way to higher status.

As a model to study socially-generated stress, Sapolsky has argued, baboons are very useful, not least as you don't have to consider any of the other factors which affect humans, given none of them smoke or drink, or are overweight, and they all have exactly the same diet. They even usually face few physical stressors beyond the occasional drought. In a typical day, they spend around three hours finding food, leaving, as Sapolsky puts it, 'nine hours of daylight for them to be really crappy to the other baboons'.[28]

However useful a model, baboons are just one example of how stress can operate. Other research has shown that in species like African wild dogs and ring-tailed lemurs, dominant animals show the highest cortisol levels, most likely because they have to maintain their dominance through repeated fighting.

Also, cultures can change. One troop of baboons studied by Sapolsky was ravaged by an outbreak of tuberculosis which killed half the males, including most of the more aggressive animals. The remaining troop became less hierarchical, with higher levels of mutual grooming and less stress. A decade later, even when the entire population of male baboons had been replaced – in adolescence males leave the troop in which they were born – this culture remained.

For one final example, let us look to a much less well-known but perhaps even more extraordinary animal, particularly in the way it handles stress: the naked mole-rat. Native to east Africa, these rodents are usually less than 10cm long. With hairless bodies covered in pink, heavily creased folds of skin, and gigantic, protruding incisors, they have been described as resembling either a tiny walrus or a cocktail sausage with teeth. They are the longest-lived of all rodents, surviving over thirty years in captivity and even more in the wild. When they dig deep into sand to create their complex burrow systems, they can survive for five hours with only 5 per cent oxygen and for eighteen minutes with no oxygen at all. Their bodies also seem to barely deteriorate with age.

But this is just the start of their interest to researchers. Naked mole-rats live in a way that is known as eusociality – the highest level of social organization, involving things like mutual care and a division of labour. It is seen in insects like ants, bees and termites, and a few types of shrimps. With mammals, it exists only in humans. And naked mole-rats.

Colonies of the creatures are more socially regulated than a nineteenth-century European royal court. There is a queen, who is notably bigger, and a handful of male consorts, with every other mole-rat being subordinate. Numbering anything up to 200 or so, these subordinates do not reproduce and have clearly defined supportive roles, such as 'soldiers' who defend the colony, food gatherers and burrowers.

In tests, the mole rats' cortisol levels rose noticeably if they were removed from the colony, but when they were amid their own structures there was no apparent relationship between hierarchy and cortisol. Neither being dominant nor submissive seemed to be a stressor.[29]

So, other than being a fascinating diversion into the slightly niche world of psychobiology, what do all these complex and much-shifting animal-world situations tell us about how, as humans, we can think about stress? Most obviously, they take us back to the universal maxim of stress intimated from the start of the chapter: it never exists in a vacuum, and so neither do the answers. These will always be different for each person, and even for an individual they will often evolve over time. For one person, the best option might be several years of psychotherapy to untangle a childhood predilection to surges in cortisol. For another, finding a new job or undertaking twenty minutes a day of mindfulness or yoga might have some impact. Or else the stresses might be so obviously unfixable that the best option is to take up gentle running or get off the bus a few stops early to walk some of the way to work.

Finally, for some, none of these may seem realistic, at least for now. Not everyone can (or should) be the human equivalent of what Robert Sapolsky calls a 'watering-hole-half-full' baboon. But that does not represent a defeat. Sometimes one of the best responses a person can have to stress is to stop, think for a while, and realize that they are stressed. If you can pinpoint a reason why, all the better. But these reasons can be elusive and deep-rooted, hiding just out of sight.

And there is one lesson we can all take from the various creatures which have populated this chapter. It is impossible to emulate them by not anticipating or brooding on life's pressures. But a rat, a baboon and especially a naked mole-rat, never feels guilty about stress. And neither should we.

Epilogue

A Light in the Mist

When you tell someone you are writing a book about stress, the questions come thick and fast. How do you know you're stressed? What can you do about it? Is it really as big a problem as presented? Then there are the more specific queries.

One asked several times is why we seem to fall ill as soon as a particularly stressful period has finished, for example a major project at work, a big family event, or exams – a phenomenon known as 'the let-down effect'. The answer has several parts. It can simply be a factor of the way stress affects the immune system; while chronic stress undermines it, shorter-term stress can boost the way it works. But there is an equally valid counter-theory: we don't actually get ill when a big event is over, we just happen to notice it. If you start to develop a cold two days before an exam or a wedding, the chances are you will be so distracted that you won't pay it any attention – that only happens once the mental foreground has cleared. Also, it could simply be confirmation bias – the general idea of the let-down effect is sufficiently well-known that people tend to remember when they fall ill post-stress, and not when they don't.

Another area which prompted a lot of queries if, and how, stress can affect different people in different ways. And as we have seen, the answer to 'if' is a very definite yes, taking in both individual circumstances and wider things like gender, ethnicity and whether or not you are able-bodied. The latter can often become relevant in ways that lead to the idea known as intersectionality, which tries to understand how different types of disadvantage and bias, or the opposite, mingle together. To take an example from Chapter 10, in terms of the statistical chances of being susceptible to stress, Kate had the inbuilt advantage of relative economic privilege but also faced the negatives of being a woman and – as much as one consultation could gauge – having faced an upbringing with some difficulties. Similarly, Yusuf in Chapter 7 had money, professional status and some control over his workload, but also a greater chance he would experience stress due to his ethnicity, plus the physiological add-on that this was more likely to lead to type 2 diabetes.

Some of what you might term the structural impacts of stress are so normalized and in-built that we barely notice them. One of the most fascinating examples is the way it apparently contributes to the greater likelihood of women feeling cold in their hands and feet. In general body-thermostat terms, men tend to have a higher metabolic rate, up to 20 per cent greater than women. A by-product of burning more bodily fuel to keep your system ticking over is that you stay warmer. Compounding this is the very non-biological fact that thermostats in many public buildings are set according to a historic model based on men's metabolic rates. But when it comes to the extremities, fight-or-flight also plays a role. Among the several physiological changes instigated by the influx of hormones when faced with a cause of stress is a rush of blood towards your organs and major muscles, preparing you to deal with whatever peril is presented. This, incidentally, is also why people's faces can often go pale when they are in danger. But as well as taking blood away from your face, it takes it from your hands and feet. This process appears to be more finely-attuned in women than in men, meaning that even if there is no other stress, cold temperatures alone can trigger the effect to a greater extent in women. Hence the higher chance of colder hands and feet, and an entire sub-industry which markets ultra-warm gloves and thick, fleecy socks primarily at women.

When it comes to stress as an overall problem, the more you understand how it works, the more you notice its effects – and just about everywhere. Take one example, briefly mentioned earlier: the growing number of people who are unable to work due to long-term ill health.

More or less every reason raised as a possible factor for this has echoes in what we have seen across this book.

One is the fast-rising number of younger people in particular who are unable to work due to mental health conditions like anxiety and depression, which have a very close connection to stress. A report by the UK's Resolution Foundation think-tank concluded that young British people, those aged eighteen to twenty-four, were the most likely age group to experience mental health problems. Two decades earlier, they were the least likely.[1] There are all sorts of possible reasons, including young people being at the sharp end of the Covid pandemic. But one intriguing factor could be the fact that people now coming into adulthood grew up amid notable economic turmoil, both from the 2008 global crash and recession, and, in the UK, with the political choices of austerity from 2010 onwards. Being unable to pay a bill, as we have seen, is a major stress which can impact everyone in a household, including infants and children.

By this metric, we could expect worse to come, as the children of austerity grow up. Such economic pressures also include housing, another area where the UK fares badly. While the number of people sleeping rough remains relatively low, an astonishing 1 in 200 households now live in insecure emergency accommodation, something which creates vast amounts of stress.

Many other people who are unable to work are in this position because of long-term physical ill health, often connected to type 2 diabetes and obesity. And while these very much exist outside of stress, too, there is overwhelming evidence that stress makes both conditions more widespread and more acute, and that both in turn are major drivers of more stress.

This is at risk of becoming a slightly gloomy coda to the book. So let us bring the focus back to the personal, with another recurrent question: how do you know if you are stressed? As stated already, the only person who will know this is the person affected. Yes, there are tests for cortisol and blood glucose, or other proxies like blood pressure. But they give only a partial picture, and at one remove. If you *feel* stressed, then you *are* stressed, even if someone tries to tell you either that you are not, or that you should not be.

Another point to note is that people very often don't realize that they are stressed, or at least not quite how stressed they really are. Stress is the epitome of the 'boiled frog' analogy, which says that a frog put directly into boiling water will leap out, but one that goes into in cool water which is gradually heated will allow itself to be poached to death. This is, in two senses, not literally the case: a frog would almost certainly die immediately if plunged into boiling water, and would also jump out if the water it was in became hot. But as an analogy, it is resonant. Stress can very easily build up and become normalized, particularly given the way it tends to create the tunnel-vision mindset we saw in Chapter 5, leaving no space for wider contemplation.

One of the most powerful ways that psychotherapy can help with stress is to provide a neutral, quiet space in which the most simple and fundamental of questions – 'How do you feel?' – can be asked and examined. But the same can be done in a less formal setting. It could be a friend, a partner, a child, a parent, even a co-worker or, occasionally, a stranger asking this. Very often, of course, people already know they are stressed, or come to the realization alone.

If you have picked up this book, and particularly if you have made it this close to the end, there is a fairly strong chance that you have an interest in stress. It might be curiosity, or interest in the way it manifests unequally. It might, instead, be to better understand the predicament of a loved one. Whatever your circumstances, but particularly if you have read our words either because you already knew that you were stressed or because you now realize this, do remember that this first step – *Yes, I am stressed* – can be one of the most important to take. A defining characteristic of stress is that it can feel overwhelming. But much of this is because of its formlessness, the way it wraps itself around a life without you even realizing this has happened.

Even when shared, stress can feel very lonely, as we saw from the struggles Deborah and her partner went through to conceive, outlined in Chapter 8, a joint experience which nonetheless almost pushed them apart. It can also feel endless.

This book is not a solution to any stress felt by you or anyone else in your life. It might have provided some ideas about possible routes out. Perhaps it just helped you understand whatever is causing the stress, or the circumstances that make you feel it, whether or not anything can be done, immediately or longer-term. Stress can feel like a mist surrounding you. With luck, at least one chapter, hopefully more, will have sent a shaft of light through this murkiness, if not necessarily lighting the way forward then at least giving a better clue as to where you are now.

Whatever the situation, do remember: this is not a weakness, or a failing, let alone an individual one. There are much, much bigger factors at work. Stress is all around us. In many ways it is intrinsic to life. But it does not, or at least should not, define us.

Acknowledgements

Peter

My first thanks has to be to Richard, who came up with the initial idea for a truly modern book on stress, and whose expertise, research and work provided its bedrock.

Many thanks also to everyone who talked to me about all aspects of stress and its history and consequences, from the perils of the modern workplace to the discovery of its link to status and control.

I am always hugely grateful to Rachel Mills, my amazing agent, for her ideas, enthusiasm and encouragement. And, very obviously, thanks to Jodie Lancet-Grant and Cara Waudby-Tolley for signing us up to Bluebird and for having such good ideas for how the book could be improved.

This book was written in snatches of time off from my day job with *The Guardian*'s political team, and I couldn't work with a better, more supportive or lovelier bunch of people: Pippa Crerar, Jessica Elgot, Rowena Mason, John Crace, Aletha Adu, Kiran Stacey, Eleni Courea, Andrew Sparrow, Ben Quinn and Ellie Cole.

Finally: thank you to Jane for giving her always thoughtful and hugely useful views on everything from the sample chapter to the finished book, and to Ralph and Robin for . . . well, for helping me feel less stressed. Most of the time.

Richard

I would like to thank Peter for believing in the ideas behind this book and supporting it from the start. You turned a daunting prospect into an enjoyable experience. Thanks also to Rachel Mills for all her support and enthusiasm.

I would also like thank Professor David James at Sydney University. Despite the geographical distance between us, he has always been supportive of my research career. David also added his knowledge to the paragraphs on protein kinases.

I would also like to thank two individuals who very much helped me to get to where I am today – both professionally and personally. These are Doctors Neil Maxwell and Peter Watt. Thank you to you both for all your support and guidance.

Much of my clinical work in insulin resistance has taken me down many other avenues. One of these has been fertility, and for this I would like to thank Dr Giada Frontino. Giada is not only a fantastic doctor, but a great person, and I am truly grateful for her input on fertility both in this book and more generally. I would also like to say a big thanks to Dr Ralph Rogers for being the person he is. You have done a lot for me over the years, and I will be forever grateful. Lastly to my son Avery. Despite everything you have been through, your default to life is to smile. A lesser person would have given up. A great deal of the motivation for this book has come from you and I am extremely proud to be your father.

Notes

CHAPTER 1: A NEW UNDERSTANDING OF STRESS

1. 'Stress: Are we coping?' Report by the Mental Health Foundation.
2. 'UK Labour Market: February 2024', Office for National Statistics labour market (13 February 2024).
3. McEwen, Bruce, 'The neurobiology of stress: from serendipity to clinical relevance.' *Brain Research* (2000), 886 (1–2): 172–89. Bruce McEwen is a US neuroendocrinologist – someone who studies the interactions between hormones and the brain.
4. Selye, Hans, 'A syndrome produced by diverse nocuous agents', *Nature* (1936), 138: 32.
5. Marmot, Michael, *The Health Gap: Challenge of an Unequal World*, Bloomsbury (2015), p. 2.
6. This has been noted by several researchers, including Michael Marmot. The statistic originates from the London Public Health Observatory.
7. From the Office for National Statistics. The most recent data showed the life-expectancy for women. 'Health state life expectancies in England, Northern Ireland and Wales: between 2011 to 2013 and 2020 to 2022'. https://www.ons.gov.uk/peoplepopulationandcommunity/healthandsocialcare/healthandlifeexpectancies/bulletins/healthstatelifeexpectanciesuk/between2011to2013and2020to2022
8. Mani, A., Mullainathan, S., Shafir, E. et al., 'Poverty impedes cognitive function', *Science* (2013), Aug 30;341(6149):976–80.
9. Ibid.
10. Gianaros, P. J., Horenstein, J. A., Hariri, A. R. et al., 'Potential neural embedding of parental social standing.' *Soc Cogn Affect Neurosci.* 2008 Jun;3(2):91–6.

11 Ku, M., Kim, J., Won, J. E. et al., 'Smart, soft contact lens for wireless immunosensing of cortisol.' *Sci Adv.* 2020 Jul 8;6(28).

CHAPTER 2: A SHORT HISTORY OF STRESS

1   Selye, Hans, *The Stress of Life*, McGraw Hill (1978), p. 17.
2   Selye, Hans and McKeown, Thomas, 'Studies on the physiology of the maternal placenta in the rat', *Proceedings of the Royal Society of London* (1935), 119: 1–31.
3   Selye, Hans, 'A syndrome produced by diverse nocuous agents', *Nature* (1936), 138: 32.
4   Rosch, Paul J., 'Reminiscences of Hans Selye, and the birth of "stress".' *International Journal of Emergency Mental Health.* (1999), Winter;1(1): 59–66. PMID: 11227756.
5   Selye, *The Stress of Life*, op. cit., p. 52.
6   Beard, George Miller, *American Nervousness: Its Causes and Consequences*, Putnam (1881).
7   *Diagnostic and Statistical Manual of Mental Disorders* (second edition), American Psychiatric Association (1968).
8   Stewart, D. N. and de R. Winser, D. M., 'Incidence of perforated peptic ulcer: effect of heavy air raids', *Lancet* (1942), 1: 259–61.
9   Spicer, C. C., Stewart, D. N. and de R. Winser, D. M., 'Perforated peptic ulcer during the period of heavy air-raids', *Lancet* (1944), 243(6279).
10 Jones, E., '"The gut war": Functional somatic disorders in the UK during the Second World War', History of the Human Sciences (2012), 25(5): 30–48.
11 Letter from Hans Selye, *Lancet* (1943), 241(6234).
12 Roberts, Ffrangcon, 'Stress and the General Adaptation Syndrome', *British Medical Journal* (1950), 2(4670): 104–5.
13 Jackson, Mark, *The Age of Stress: Science and the Search for Stability*, Oxford University Press (2013).
14 Preston, Frank, *Healthy Minds and Bodies: Your Guide in All Medical, Marriage and Motherhood Problems*, Waverley (1956).
15 Selye, *The Stress of Life*, op. cit.
16 Ibid.
17 Selye, Hans, *Stress Without Distress*, Lippincott Williams & Wilkins (1974).
18 Toffler, Alvin, *Future Shock*, Random House (1970).
19 *Future Shock*, directed by Alex Grasshoff and narrated by Orson Welles (1972).

20 American Institute of Stress, 'Our History', https://www.stress.org/our-history
21 Friedman, Meyer and Rosenman, Ray H., *Type A Behaviour and Your Heart*, Random House (1974).
22 Petticrew, M. P. and Lee, K., 'The "Father of Stress" meets "Big Tobacco": Hans Selye and the tobacco industry', *American Journal of Public Health* (2011), 101(3): 411–18.
23 Ibid.
24 Holmes, T. H. and Rahe, R. H., 'The Social Readjustment Rating Scale', *Journal of Psychosomatic Research*, 11(2): 213–18.
25 Rahe, R. H., Mahan, J. L. and Arthur, R. J., 'Prediction of near-future health change from subjects' preceding life changes', *Journal of Psychosomatic Research* (1970), 14(4): 401–6.
26 Kanner, A. D., Coyne, J. C., Schaefer, C. et al., 'Comparison of two modes of stress measurement: daily hassles and uplifts versus major life events', *Journal of Behavioral Medicine* (1981), 4(1): 1–39.
27 'Stress! Seeking Cures for Modern Anxieties', *Time* magazine (1983), 6 June.
28 Karasek, R., Baker, D., Marxer, F. et al., 'Job decision latitude, job demands, and cardiovascular disease: a prospective study of Swedish men', *American Journal of Public Health* (1981), 71(7): 694–705

CHAPTER 3: THE HORMONES THAT SHAPE YOUR LIFE

1 Bayliss, W. M. and Starling, E. H., 'The mechanism of pancreatic secretion', *Journal of Physiology* (1902), 28(5): 325–53.
2 Oliver, G., 'On the therapeutic employment of the suprarenal glands', *British Medical Journal* (1895), 2(1811): 653–5.
3 Schawrcz, J., 'Getting "Steinached" was all the rage in Roaring '20s', Office for Science and Society (2017), McGill University, 20 March, https://www.mcgill.ca/oss/article/health-history-science-science-everywhere/getting-steinached-was-all-rage-roaring-20s
4 Ibid.
5 Berman, Louis, *New Creations in Human Beings*, Doubleday, Doran and Co. (1938).
6 Kendall, Edward, *Cortisone: Memoirs of a Hormone Hunter*, Macmillan (1972).
7 Cushing, Harvey, *The Pituitary Body and Its Disorders: Clinical States Produced by Disorders of the Hypophysis Cerebri*, J. B. Lippincott Company (1912).

8 O'Byrne, N. A., Yuen, F., Butt, W. Z. et al., 'Sleep and circadian regulation of cortisol: a short review', Current Opinion in Endocrine and Metabolic Research (2021), 18: 178–86.

9 Zuraikat F. M. et al., 'Chronic Insufficient sleep in women impairs insulin sensitivity independent of adiposity changes: results of a randomized trial', Diabetes Care (2024), Jan 1;47(1) https://pubmed.ncbi.nlm.nih.gov/37955852/

10 Vedhara, K., Hyde, J., Gilchrist, I. D. et al., 'Acute stress, memory, attention and cortisol', Psychoneuroendocrinology (2000) 25(6): 535–49.

11 Schmidt, S. C. E., Gnam, J. P., Kopf, M. et al., 'The influence of cortisol, flow, and anxiety on performance in e-sports: a field study', Biomed Research International (2020): 9651245.

12 Weiss, J. M., 'Somatic effects of predictable and unpredictable shock', Psychosomatic Medicine (1970), 32(4): 397–408.

13 Deinzer, R., Kirschbaum, C., Gresele, C. et al., 'Adrenocortical responses to repeated parachute jumping and subsequent h-CRH challenge in inexperienced healthy subjects', Physiology and Behavior (1997), 61(4): 507–11.

14 Pulopulos, M. M., Baeken, C. and De Raedt, R, 'Cortisol response to stress: the role of expectancy and anticipatory stress regulation', Hormones and Behavior (2020), 117: 104587.

CHAPTER 4: THE NEED FOR HOMEOSTASIS

1 Bernard, Claude, *Leçons sur les phénomènes de la vie communs aux animaux et aux végétaux*, J.-B. Baillière (1878).

2 Cannon, Walter B., *The Wisdom of the Body*, W. W. Norton and Company (1932).

3 Mainous, A. G. III, Tanner, R. J., Baker, R. et al., 'Prevalence of prediabetes in England from 2003 to 2011: population-based, cross-sectional study. BMJ Open. 2014 Jun 9;4(6):e005002. doi: 10.1136/bmjopen-2014-005002. PMID: 24913327; PMCID: PMC4054625.

4 Cannon, Walter B., *Bodily Changes in Pain, Hunger, Fear, and Rage: An Account of Recent Researches into the Function of Emotional Excitement*, D. Appleton and Company (1915).

5 Cannon, Walter B., *The Wisdom of the Body*, W. W. Norton and Company (1932).

6 Langdon-Brown, W., *The Integration of the Endocrine System*, Cambridge: Cambridge University Press (1935).

7 Wade, Nicholas, *The Nobel Duel*, Anchor Press/Doubleday (1981).

8   Hanson, M. D. and Chen. E., 'Daily stress, cortisol, and sleep: the moderating role of childhood psychosocial environments', *Health Psychology* (2010), 29(4): 394–402.

9   Dettling, A. C., Gunnar, M. R. and Donzella, B., 'Cortisol levels of young children in full-day childcare centers: relations with age and temperament', *Psychoneuroendocrinology* (1999), 24(5): 519–36.

10 Bauer M. E., Jeckel C. M. and Luz C., 'The role of stress factors during aging of the immune system', *Ann N Y Acad Sci.* (2009), Feb;1153: 139–52.
    Oei N. Y., Everaerd W. T., Elzinga B. M., van Well S. and Bermond B., 'Psychosocial stress impairs working memory at high loads: an association with cortisol levels and memory retrieval', *Stress* (2006), Sep;9(3): 133–41. Ouanes S., Popp J., 'High Cortisol and the Risk of Dementia and Alzheimer's Disease: A Review of the Literature', *Front Aging Neurosci.* (2019), Mar 1;11:43.

11 Rizza, R. A., Mandarino, L. J. and Gerich, J. E., 'Cortisol-induced insulin resistance in man: impaired suppression of glucose production and stimulation of glucose utilization due to a postreceptor detect of insulin action', *Journal of Clinical Endocrinology and Metabolism* (1982), 54(1): 131–8.

12 McEwen, B. S. and Stellar, E., 'Stress and the individual. Mechanisms leading to disease', *Archives of Internal Medicine* (1993), 153(18): 2093–101.

13 Hermann, R., Biallas, B., Predel, H. G. et al., 'Physical versus psychosocial stress: effects on hormonal, autonomic, and psychological parameters in healthy young men', *Stress* (2019), 22(1): 103–12.

14 Hill, E. E., Zack, E., Battaglini, C. et al., 'Exercise and circulating cortisol levels: the intensity threshold effect', *Journal of Endocrinological Investigation* (2008), 31: 587–91.

15 Dote-Montero, M., Carneiro-Barrera, A., Martinez-Vizcaino, V. et al., 'Acute effect of HIIT on testosterone and cortisol levels in healthy individuals: a systematic review and meta-analysis', *Scandinavian Journal of Medicine and Science in Sports* (2021), 31(9): 1722–44.

16 Hackney, A. C. and Walz, E. A., 'Hormonal adaptation and the stress of exercise training: the role of glucocorticoids', *Trends in Sport Sciences* (2013): 20(4).

17 Borrega-Mouquinho, Y., Sánchez-Gómez, J., Fuentes-García, J. P. et al., 'Effects of high-intensity interval training and moderate-intensity training on stress, depression, anxiety, and resilience in healthy adults during Coronavirus Disease 2019 confinement: a randomized controlled trial', *Frontiers in Psychology* (2021), 12: 643069.

CHAPTER 5: STRESS, STATUS AND WORK

1. Health and Safety at Work Act 1974.
2. Kirby, J., 'The stress of work and work of stress in Britain in the late twentieth century', *Contemporary British History* (2022), 36(4): 622–45.
3. 'Working Can Be a Health Hazard', *Sunday Times*, 24 February 1985.
4. 'Stress in America 2023: a nation recovering from collective trauma', *American Psychological Association* (2023), https://www.apa.org/news/press/releases/stress/2023/collective-trauma-recovery
5. 'UK Labour Market: February 2024', Office for National Statistics labour market (13 February 2024).
6. Sapolsky, R. M., 'Glucocorticoids, the evolution of the stress-response, and the primate predicament', *Neurobiology of Stress* (2021), 20(14): 100320.
7. Thomson, D., 'Civil Service Sick Leave' (1967).
8. Marmot, M. G., Shipley, M. J. and Rose, G., 'Inequalities in death – specific explanations of a general pattern?', *Lancet* (1984), 1(8384): 1003–6.
9. Marmot, M. G., Smith, G. D., Stansfeld, S., Patel, C., North, F., Head, J., White, I., Brunner, E. and Feeney, A., 'Health inequalities among British civil servants: the Whitehall II study', *Lancet* (1991) Jun 8;337(8754): 1387–93.
10. In conversation with the author.
11. Hertzman, C., 'The significance of early childhood adversity', *Paediatrics & Child Health* (2013), 18(3): 127–8.
12. Hart, B. and Risley, T. R., 'American parenting of language-learning children: persisting differences in family–child interactions observed in natural home environments', *Developmental Psychology* (1992), 28(6): 1096–105.
13. Hertzman, 'The significance of early childhood adversity', op. cit.
14. Shih, M., Pittinsky, T. L. and Ambady, N., 'Stereotype susceptibility: identity salience and shifts in quantitative performance', *Psychological Science* (1999), 10(1): 80–83.
15. Henry, P. J., Reyna, C. and Weiner, B., 'Hate welfare but help the poor: how the attributional content of stereotypes explains the paradox of reactions to the destitute in America', *Journal of Applied Social Psychology* (2004), 34(1), 34–58.
16. Cozzarelli, Catherine, Wilkinson, Anna V. and Tagler, Michael J., 'Attitudes toward the poor and attributions for poverty', *Journal of Social Issues* (2001), 57(2): 207–27.
17. Joseph Rowntree Foundation, 'Anxiety nation? Economic insecurity and mental distress in 2020s Britain', November 2022.

18 Costello, E. J., Compton, S. N. and Keeler, G., 'Relationships between poverty and psychopathology: a natural experiment', *JAMA* (2003), 290(15): 2023–9.
19 'Health Survey for England 2021, Part 3: Drinking Alcohol', NHS (December 2022), https://digital.nhs.uk/data-and-information/publications/statistical/health-survey-for-england/2021/part-3-drinking-alcohol#chapter-index
20 Shah, A. K., Mullainathan, S. and Shafir, E., 'Some consequences of having too little', *Science* (2012), 338(6107): 682–5.
21 Mani, A., Mullainathan, S., Shafir E. et al., 'Poverty impedes cognitive function', *Science* (2013), 341(6149): 976–80.
22 Shiels, P. G. et al., 'Accelerated telomere attrition is associated with relative household income, diet and inflammation in the pSoBid cohort', *PLoS One* (2011), 6(7): e22521.
23 Lin, J. and Epel, E., 'Stress and telomere shortening: insights from cellular mechanisms', *Ageing Research Reviews* (2022), 73: 101507.
24 Ramazzini, B., *De morbis artificum diatriba* (1713).
25 Hill, J. and Trist, E., 'Temporary withdrawal from work under full employment. The formation of an absence culture' (1955), *Human Relations*, 8: 121–52.
26 Glass, D. C., Reim, B. and Singer, J. E., 'Behavioural consequences of adaptation to controllable and uncontrollable noise', *Journal of Experimental Social Psychology* (1971), 7(2), 244–257.
27 Hanson, J. D., Larson, M. E. and Snowdon, C. T., 'The effects of control over high intensity noise on plasma cortisol levels in rhesus monkeys', *Behavioral Biology* (1976), 16(3): 333–40.
28 Walker, Peter, 'Call centre staff to be monitored via webcam for home-working "infractions"', *Guardian* (26 March 2021).

CHAPTER 6: CARBOHYDRATES, APPETITES AND STIGMA: STRESS AND WEIGHT

1 Filgueiras, M. S., Pessoa, M. C., Bressan, J. et al., 'Characteristics of the obesogenic environment around schools are associated with body fat and low-grade inflammation in Brazilian children', *Public Health Nutrition* (2023), 26(11): 2407–17.
2 Baker, C., 'Obesity statistics', UK Parliament: House of Commons Library (2023), https://commonslibrary.parliament.uk/research-briefings/sn03336/
3 Hadjiolova, I., Mintcheva, L., Dunev, S. et al., 'Physical working capacity in obese women after an exercise programme for body

weight reduction', *International Journal of Obesity* (1982), 6(4): 405–10.

4   Rodríguez-Sureda, V., López-Tejero, M. D., Llobera, M. et al., 'Social stress profoundly affects lipid metabolism: over-expression of SR-BI in liver and changes in lipids and lipases in plasma and tissues of stressed mice', *Atherosclerosis* (2007), 195(1): 57–65

5   Epel, E. S., McEwen, B., Seeman, T. et al., 'Stress and body shape: stress-induced cortisol secretion is consistently greater among women with central fat', *Psychosomatic Medicine* (2000) 62(5): 623–32.

6   Wallis, D. J. and Hetherington, M. M., 'Stress and eating: the effects of ego-threat and cognitive demand on food intake in restrained and emotional eaters', *Appetite* (2004), 43(1): 39–46.

7   Noppe, G., van den Akker, E. L., de Rijke, Y. B. et al., 'Long-term glucocorticoid concentrations as a risk factor for childhood obesity and adverse body-fat distribution', *International Journal of Obesity* (2016), 40(10): 1503–9.

8   Kouvonen, A., Stafford, M., De Vogli, R. et al., 'Negative aspects of close relationships as a predictor of increased body mass index and waist circumference: the Whitehall II study', *American Journal of Public Health* (2011), 101(8): 1474–80.

9   Rogers, P. J., Vural. Y., Berridge-Burley, N. et al., 'Evidence that carbohydrate-to-fat ratio and taste, but not energy density or NOVA level of processing, are determinants of food liking and food reward', *Appetite* (2024), 193: 107124.

10 Rehkamp, S., 'A look at calorie sources in the American diet', US Department of Agriculture Economic Research Service (5 December 2016), https://www.ers.usda.gov/amber-waves/2016/december/a-look-at-calorie-sources-in-the-american-diet

11 UK Department for Environment, Food & Rural Affairs: *Food Statistics Pocketbook, 2013*.

12 Brown, R. E., Sharma, A. M., Ardern, C. I. et al., 'Secular differences in the association between caloric intake, macronutrient intake, and physical activity with obesity', *Obesity Research and Clinical Practice* (2016): 10(3): 243–55.

13 Armstrong, A., Jungbluth Rodriguez, K., Sabag, A. et al., 'Effect of aerobic exercise on waist circumference in adults with overweight or obesity: A systematic review and meta-analysis', *Obesity Reviews* (2022), 23(8): e13446.

CHAPTER 7: THE TIDAL WAVE OF ILLNESS – STRESS AND DIABETES

1. Statistics from the International Diabetes Federation, https://idf.org/news/new-diabetes-estimates/
2. Magliano, D. J. and Boyko, E. J., *IDF Diabetes Atlas* (tenth edition), (2021)
3. Willis, T., 'Pharmaceutice rationalis, sive diatriba de medicamentorum operationibus in humano corpore' (1679).
4. Karamanou, M., Protogerou, A., Tsoucalas, G. et al., 'Milestones in the history of diabetes mellitus: the main contributors', *World Journal of Diabetes* (2016), 7(1): 1–7.
5. Tattersall, Robert, *Diabetes: The Biography*, Oxford University Press (2009).
6. Banting, F. G., Best, C. H., Collip, J. B. et al., 'Pancreatic extracts in the treatment of diabetes mellitus', *Canadian Medical Association Journal* (1922), 12: 141–6.
7. Tattersall, *Diabetes*, op. cit.
8. Manousaki, D., Kent, Jack W. Jr., Haack, K. et al., 'TBC1D4 disruption is common among the Inuit and leads to underdiagnosis of Type 2 diabetes', *Diabetes Care* (2016) 39(11): 1889–95.
9. Chandola T., Brunner, E. and Marmot M., 'Chronic stress at work and the metabolic syndrome: prospective study', *British Medical Journal* (2006), 332(7540): 521–5.
10. Virk, J., Li, J., Vestergaard, M. et al., 'Prenatal exposure to bereavement and type-2 diabetes: a Danish longitudinal population based study', *PLoS One* (2012), 7(8): e43508.
11. Novak, M., Björck, L., Giang K. W. et al., 'Perceived stress and incidence of type 2 diabetes: a 35-year follow-up study of middle-aged Swedish men', *Diabetic Medicine* (2013), 30(1), e8–16.

CHAPTER 8: THE DELICATE BALANCE: HOW STRESS CAN AFFECT FERTILITY

1. Karunyam, B. V., Abdul Karim, A. K., Naina Mohamed, I. et al., 'Infertility and cortisol: a systematic review', *Frontiers in Endocrinology* (2023), 14: 1147306.
2. Ibid.
3. Joseph, D. N. and Whirledge, S., 'Stress and the HPA axis: balancing homeostasis and fertility', *International Journal of Molecular Sciences* (2017), 18(10): 2224.

4 Massey, A. J., Campbell, B. K., Raine-Fenning, N. et al., 'Relationship between hair and salivary cortisol and pregnancy in women undergoing IVF', *Psychoneuroendocrinology* (2016) 74: 397–405.
5 Csemiczky, G., Landgren, B. M. and Collins, A., 'The influence of stress and state anxiety on the outcome of IVF-treatment: psychological and endocrinological assessment of Swedish women entering IVF-treatment', *Acta obstetricia et gynecologica Scandinavica* (2000), 79(2): 113–18.
6 Vartiainen, H., Saarikoski, S., Halonen, P. et al., 'Psychosocial factors, female fertility and pregnancy: a prospective study – Part I: Fertility', *Journal of Psychosomatic Obstetrics and Gynaecology* (1994), 15(2): 67–75.
7 Lampiao, F., 'Variation of semen parameters in healthy medical students due to exam stress', *Malawi Medical Journal* (2009), 21(4): 166–7.
8 Abu-Musa, A. A., Nassar, A. H., Hannoun, A. B. et al., 'Effect of the Lebanese civil war on sperm parameters', *Fertility and Sterility* (2007), 88(6): 1579–82.
9 DeStefano, F., Annest, J. L., Kresnow, M. J. et al., 'Semen characteristics of Vietnam veterans', *Reproductive Toxicology* (1989), 3(3): 165–73.
10 Fenster, L., Katz, D. F., Wyrobek, A. J. et al., 'Effects of psychological stress on human semen quality', *Journal of Andrology* (1997) 18(2): 194–202.
11 Fukuda, M., Fukuda, K., Shimizu, T. et al., 'Kobe earthquake and reduced sperm motility', *Human Reproduction* (1996), 11(6): 1244–6.
12 Dobson, R., 'Fewer boys born in New York after 9/11 attacks', *British Medical Journal* (2006), 333(7567): 516.
13 Masukume, G., Ryan, M., Masukume, R. et al., 'COVID-19 induced birth sex ratio changes in England and Wales', *PeerJ* (2023), 11: e14618.
14 Zorn, B., Šućur, V., Stare, J. et al., 'Decline in sex ratio at birth after 10-day war in Slovenia: brief communication', *Human Reproduction* (2002), 17(12): 3173–7.
15 Bale, P., Doust, J. and Dawson, D., 'Gymnasts, distance runners, anorexics body composition and menstrual status', *Journal of Sports Medicine and Physical Fitness* (1996) 36(1): 49–53.
16 O'Loughlin, J. I., Rellini, A. H. and Brotto, L. A., 'How does childhood trauma impact women's sexual desire? Role of depression, stress, and cortisol', *Journal of Sex Research* (2020), 57(7): 836–47.
17 Hamilton, L. D., Rellini, A. H., Meston, C. M., 'Cortisol, sexual arousal, and affect in response to sexual stimuli', *Journal of Sexual Medicine* (2008) 5(9): 2111–18. Erratum in *Journal of Sexual Medicine* (2008), 5(11): 2735.

CHAPTER 9: LOVE, TOUCH AND INHERITANCE: EARLY YEARS AND STRESS

1. Barker, D. J., Winter, P. D., Osmond, C. et al., 'Weight in infancy and death from ischaemic heart disease', *Lancet* (1989), 2(8663): 577–80.
2. Ding, X., Liang, M., Wu, Y. et al., 'The impact of prenatal stressful life events on adverse birth outcomes: a systematic review and meta-analysis', *Journal of Affective Disorders* (2021), 287: 406–16.
3. Barker, D. J., Osmond, C. and Pannett, B., 'Why Londoners have low death rates from ischaemic heart disease and stroke', *British Medical Journal* (1992), 305(6868): 1551–4.
4. Levine S., Chevalier, J. A. and Korchin, S. J., 'The effects of early shock and handling on later avoidance learning', *Journal of Personality* (1956), 24(4): 475–93.
5. Weaver, I., Cervoni, N., Champagne, F. et al., 'Epigenetic programming by maternal behavior', *Nature Neuroscience* (2004), 7: 847–54 (2004).
6. Harlow, H. F., 'The nature of love', *American Psychologist* (1958), 13(12): 673–85.
7. Felitti, V. J., Anda, R. F., Nordenberg, D. et al., 'Relationship of childhood abuse and household dysfunction to many of the leading causes of death in adults: the Adverse Childhood Experiences (ACE) Study', *American Journal of Preventative Medicine* (1998) 14(4): 245–58.
8. Ibid.
9. Watson, J. B., 'Psychology as the behaviorist views it', *Psychological Review* (1913), 20(2): 158–77.
10. Speech by Granville Stanley Hall to teachers in Chicago in 1899. Quoted in: Young, J. L. (2016). G. Stanley Hall, Child Study, and the American Public. *The Journal of Genetic Psychology.* 177(6), 195–208.
11. Luther Emmett Holt, *The Care and Feeding of Children: A Catechism for the Use of Mothers and Children's Nurses*, D. Appleton and Company (1894).
12. Bowlby, J., 'The influence of early environment in the development of neurosis and neurotic character', *International Journal of Psychoanalysis* (1940), 21: 154–78.
13. Bowlby, John and Robertson, James, *A Two Year Old Goes to Hospital: A Scientific Film*, Robertson Films (1953).
14. Bowlby, John, *A Secure Base: Parent–Child Attachment and Healthy Human Development*, Basic Books (1988).
15. Ainsworth, M. D. and Bell, S. M., 'Attachment, exploration, and separation: illustrated by the behavior of one-year-olds in a strange situation', *Child Development* (1970), 41(1): 49–67.

16 Mead, M., 'A cultural anthropologist's approach to maternal deprivation', *Public Health Papers* (1962), 14: 45–62.

17 Blaffer Hrdy, Sarah, *Mothers and Others: The Evolutionary Origins of Mutual Understanding*, Harvard University Press (2011).

18 Vandell, D. L., Belsky, J., Burchinal, M. et al., 'Do effects of early child care extend to age 15 years? Results from the NICHD study of early child care and youth development', *Child Development* (2010) 81(3): 737–56.

19 Winnicott, D. W., 'Transitional objects and transitional phenomena; a study of the first not-me possession', *International Journal of Psychoanalysis* (1953), 34(2): 89–97.

20 UK government statutory maternity payment at the time of writing.

21 Isaac, A. J., Rodriguez, A., D'Anna-Hernandez, K. L. et al., 'Preschool-aged children's hair cortisol and parents' behavior, psychopathology, and stress', *Psychoneuroendocrinology* (2023), 151(6): 106052.

22 Spencer, N., Bambang, S., Logan, S. et al., 'Socioeconomic status and birth weight: comparison of an area-based measure with the Registrar General's social class', *Journal of Epidemiology and Community Health* (1999), 53(8): 495–8.

23 Tamis-LeMonda, C. S., Shannon, J. D., Cabrera, N. J. et al., 'Fathers and mothers at play with their 2- and 3-year-olds: contributions to language and cognitive development', *Child Development* (2004) 75(6): 1806–20.

24 Parenteau, A. M., Alen, N. V., Deer, L. K. et al., 'Parenting matters: parents can reduce or amplify children's anxiety and cortisol responses to acute stress', *Development and Psychopathology* (2020) 32(5): 1799–809.

25 Frankenhaeuser, M., 'Coping with stress at work', *International Journal of Health Services* (1981), 11(4): 491–510.

26 'Stress in America 2023', American Psychological Association (November 2023).

27 Tsang, A., Von Korff, M., Lee, S. et al., 'Common chronic pain conditions in developed and developing countries: gender and age differences and comorbidity with depression–anxiety disorders', *Journal of Pain* (2008), 9(10): 883–91.

28 Ruschak, I., Montéso-Curto, P., Roselló, L. et al., 'Fibromyalgia syndrome pain in men and women: a scoping review', *Healthcare* (2023) 11(2): 223.

CHAPTER 10: ROUTES OUT OF STRESS

1. Harrer, G. and Harrer, H., 'Music, emotion and autonomic function', *Music and the Brain* (1977), p. 202–16.
2. Levine, S. and Levine, R., 'Why they're not smiling: stress and discontent in the orchestral workplace', *Harmony* (1996), 2(1), 15–26.
3. Clow, A. and Smyth, N., 'Salivary cortisol as a non-invasive window on the brain' in *Stress and Brain Health: Across the Life Course*, edited by Angela Clow and Nina Smyth, *International Review of Neurobiology* (2020), 150: 1–16.
4. Drawn up by David Gordon, Professor of Social Justice at the University of Bristol, https://www.bristol.ac.uk/poverty/healthinequalities.html
5. Horwath, J., 'Stress and coping in an inner-city environment: the Cities Mentor Project coping intervention with youth living in urban poverty', College of Science and Health Theses and Dissertations, DePaul University (2021), 368.
6. Morris, J. M. et al., 'Coronary heart-disease and physical activity of work', *Lancet* (1953), 262(6795): 1053–7.
7. From research led by Dr Richard Mackenzie, as part of a collaboration, which at the time of writing is not yet published.
8. Andersen, L. B., Schnohr, P., Schroll, M. et al., 'All-cause mortality associated with physical activity during leisure time, work, sports, and cycling to work', *Archives of Internal Medicine* (2000), 160(11): 1621–8.
9. Johnson, V. W., 'The effects of music genre on spontaneous exercise and enjoyment', MSc thesis for University of Wisconsin-La Cross (2004).
10. Caplin, A., Chen, F. S., Beauchamp, M. R. et al., 'The effects of exercise intensity on the cortisol response to a subsequent acute psychosocial stressor', *Psychoneuroendocrinology* (2021), 131: 105336.
11. Allaouat, S., Halonen, J. I., Jussila, J. J. et al., 'Association between active commuting and low-grade inflammation: a population-based cross-sectional study', *European Journal of Public Health* (2024), 34(2): 292–8.
12. Shiloh, S., Sorek, G. and Terkel, J., 'Reduction of state-anxiety by petting animals in a controlled laboratory experiment', *Anxiety, Stress & Coping* (2003), 16(4), 387–95.
13. Nagengast, S. L., Baun, M. M., Megel, M. et al., 'The effects of the presence of a companion animal on physiological arousal and behavioural distress in children during a physical examination', *Journal of Pediatric Nursing* (1997) 12(6): 323–30.

14 Dreisoerner, A., Junker, N. M., Schlotz, W. et al., 'Self-soothing touch and being hugged reduce cortisol responses to stress: a randomized controlled trial on stress, physical touch, and social identity', *Comprehensive Psychoneuroendocrinology* (2021) 8: 100091.

15 Marmot, M. G. and Syme, S. L., 'Acculturation and coronary heart disease in Japanese-Americans', *American Journal of Epidemiology* (1976) 104(3): 225–47.

16 Grandner, M. A., Seixas, A., Shetty, S. et al., 'Sleep duration and diabetes risk: population trends and potential mechanisms', *Current Diabetes Reports* (2016), 16(11): 106.

17 De Nys, L., Anderson, K., Ofosu, E. F. et al., 'The effects of physical activity on cortisol and sleep: a systematic review and meta-analysis', *Psychoneuroendocrinology* (2022), 143: 105843.

18 Shively, C. A., Appt, S. E., Chen, H. et al., 'Mediterranean diet, stress resilience, and aging in nonhuman primates', *Neurobiology of Stress* (2020), 13: 100254.

19 Alufer, L., Tsaban, G., Rinott, E. et al., 'Long-term green-Mediterranean diet may favor fasting morning cortisol stress hormone; the DIRECT-PLUS clinical trial', *Frontiers in Endocrinology* (2023), 14: 1243910.

20 Tsang, C., Hodgson, L., Bussu, A. et al., 'Effect of polyphenol-rich dark chocolate on salivary cortisol and mood in adults', *Antioxidants* (2019) 8(6): 149.

21 Grupe, D. W., Stoller, J. L., Alonso, C. et al., 'The impact of mindfulness training on police officer stress, mental health, and salivary cortisol levels', *Frontiers in Psychology* (2021), 12: 720753.

22 Zaccari, B., Callahan, M. L., Storzbach, D. et al., 'Yoga for veterans with PTSD: cognitive functioning, mental health, and salivary cortisol', *Psychological Trauma* (2020), 12(8): 913–17.

23 Meier, M., Wirz, L., Dickinson, P. et al., 'Laughter yoga reduces the cortisol response to acute stress in healthy individuals', *Stress* (2021), 24(1): 44–52.

24 Hosseini, S., Heydari, A., Vakili, M. et al., 'Effect of lavender essence inhalation on the level of anxiety and blood cortisol in candidates for open-heart surgery', *Iranian Journal of Nursing and Midwifery Research* (2016), 21(4): 397–401.

25 Suyono, H., Jong, F. X. and Wijaya, S. (2020), 'Lavender, cedarwood, vetiver balm work as anti-stress treatment by reducing plasma cortisol level', *Records of Natural Products*, 8. 10–12.

26 Halo, M., Massányi, M., Mlyneková, E. et al., 'The effect of training load stress on salivary cortisol concentrations, health parameters and haematological parameters in horses', *Heliyon* (2023), 9(8): e19037.

27 Sapolsky, R. M., 'Glucocorticoids, the evolution of the stress-response, and the primate predicament', *Neurobiology of Stress* (2021), 14: 100320.
28 'Baboons, humans and stress: the cost of being an SOB', *Yale Medical Magazine* (Winter 2007).
29 Edwards, P. D., Mooney, S. J., Bosson, C. O. et al., 'The stress of being alone: removal from the colony, but not social subordination, increases fecal cortisol metabolite levels in eusocial naked mole-rats', *Hormones and Behavior* (2020) 121: 104720.

EPILOGUE

1 McCurdy, Charlie and Murphy, Louise, 'We've only just begun: Action to improve young people's mental health, education and employment', Resolution Foundation (2024).

About the Authors

Dr Richard Mackenzie is one of the UK's foremost experts on glucose metabolism, insulin resistance and their interactions with stress hormones. He is a leading researcher at the Research Centre for Health & Life Sciences (Coventry University) and the Institute of Cardio-Metabolic Medicine (University Hospital Coventry and Warwick NHS Trust). He also runs a metabolic health clinic at a distinguished London-based practice and has published more than forty journal articles, mainly on insulin resistance and diabetes.

Peter Walker is senior political correspondent with *The Guardian* and a well-known commentator and frequent broadcaster on active living and health, as well as on politics. As a journalist, he has also worked for Agence France-Presse, CNN and others, reporting from places including China, Iraq and North Korea. He has written two previous books, including *The Miracle Pill*.